Rose Colored Façade

Ivy Babbitt

To every cat I've ever loved.

Credit for the cover art goes to
Sabrina Martinez; she can be
found on Instagram at
sabby_starz

<u>Instagram Archive</u>

The following is everything I posted on my Instagram (**@sighvy_**) from 2014 to 2016. I recommend reading this section before reading the rest of the book so that you can mentally make note of where I was at throughout the story, according to the dates I posted. *(Skip to page 69 for the beginning of the story)*

Picture: half my face, one eye showing, letting people see that my skin was glowing red. **Oct 6th, 2014.**

Caption: Today was absolutely ridiculous. For the past four weeks I've been attending the first three periods of school, then doing the rest on homebound. It's a lot of walking already, but I thought I was ready to add my fourth period, which was, I thought, relatively close to my third class. There's a door right by my English class that leads outside to the portables, and I thought "Well, that's not too bad" I get outside and start to go down the long sidewalk leading to the four different areas of portables; mind you, I was wearing a sweater at the time, and it is/was 90 degrees outside. I go to the first portable which had an unreasonably long and steep ramp, check the room numbers, and see it's not even close to where I need to be. So I make my way to the next one, nearly face planting while walking down the damn ramp, and I find a classroom with an open door- the room numbers were still way off.

I asked the teacher inside where I could find 170, and she informed me that I would have to walk "all the way across the pavement towards the back parking lot, and it should be the portable right in front of the tennis court". So that walk took me about three minutes. I get there, and there's two portables; Thankfully, it was the one that DIDNT have stairs. By the time I finally got to the right classroom, my feet were dragging horribly, but I was just glad to finally be there.

I sit down and find that the class is just as great as I expected it to be, (it's a human resources class that teaches about human behavioral patterns and how to work with people, ect. I took it because I really want to become a psychologist when I'm older) the teacher was really nice. The people weren't too bad.

Things were going really well, until he told me the lunch schedule; his class has second lunch shift. This involves doing half the class, going to lunch, then going back and doing the other half. By the time I got to the cafeteria all the other students were being let out, so it was hell trying to get through the walkways. I was feeling so weak at this point that my legs were shaking, and it's not like I could get a tray, because no one was there to help me carry it, and I didn't want to bother a teacher.

So I went into the bathroom. I just wanted to cry. Im waiting to get into the handicap stall, the only one my stupid walker will fit into, and there's this girl in there; she's shouting out to someone who wasn't even there. She was just in there screaming "TERRI. TERRI! I NEED YOU TO COME IN HERE AND HELP ME. HAHAHA, DID YOU SEE SELENAS PICTURE ON INSTAGRAM" this literally went on for five minutes straight. By the time she actually got out, she looked at me, laughing, and asked "My bad, were you waiting?" I just turned around and left.

Lunch was already half over by then, so I made my way to the front entrance and called my mom on the phone, crying, telling her to pick me up. I couldn't get back to my class even if I wanted to. By the time she picked me up I was sobbing and my legs felt like they weighed fifty pounds. I'm actually getting chalices on my thumbs from the handles on my walker, and in the middle of a conversation my hands both starting cramping so badly I started crying, it lasted for two minutes.

Im exhausted. I can't stand having conversion disorder, the only person who understands is my counselor, who to my great surprise, used to have it. She got over it in six months, but for me it's been three years. Right now I honestly just feel hopeless. Sorry this is so long ☐ **#conversiondisorder #done #hopeless**

***

Picture: showing half my face (as always, back then) and my eyeliner is partially cried off, but I have a small orange flower behind my ear. **Oct 27, 2014.**

Caption: My mom picked me a flower c: so, I know my eyeliner sucks in this picture- I've been crying a lot today. I've made a decision; if I want to walk any time soon, I'm basically going to have to work my ass off until I do. That what my counselor, a former conversion disorder fighter, had to do. I'm done feeling sorry for myself. I need to just /do/ what I know needs to be done. At home, I'm going to start doing 10 minutes on the treadmill every hour, and at school I will constantly be doing things like tapping my foot, lifting my feet, ect. It's a start, I guess. Every month I'll add another minute to the treadmill time; after a month of doing 10 every hour? I'll do 11 every hour. I just want to get better. **#conversiondisorder #fighting #tired**

***

Picture: We see mom in the background holding a knife and an instruction manual; we had just opened up my brand new blue walker (snazzy!). There is a grey and white kitten sitting on top of the box it came in, and I cannot remember what its' name was for the life of me, which goes to show how dispensable animals were/are for my mother. **Oct 29, 2014.**

Caption: So, I got a new walker, and my cat got a new toy ▢ yesterday I talked with my psychologist, and I told her about my "plan" to continuously exercise until I can walk again. We had a good long talk about it, and she gave me a safer, more efficient way to look at it; I need self confidence. Not necessarily about my looks, but confidence in myself and my ability to overcome my conversion disorder. If you give two people of the exact same brain capacity the exact same test, the one who has more self confidence is more likely to pass. All my self doubt, "I can't walk", only fuels the conversion disorder further.

A study showed that it takes 21 days for your brain to process and develop a new habit. I need to, basically, rewire my brain and thought track. I'm so used to telling myself and others "I can't walk. But I /can/ walk. I simply have a harder time doing so than others, and that's okay, because it is possible to overcome conversion disorder.

So, I've decided to do a 21 day challenge- every day I'll update you guys on how I'm doing, and include one positive quote for myself and anyone else who's reading.

Day 1: "It's just a bad day; not a bad life. I did good at reminding myself "I can" and correcting myself whenever I said or thought "I can't". I got a lot of nice comments about my new walker, which was really nice c:

I did fall once, and it scared me because I thought I hurt my foot, but I got up just fine (Today is going to be short because you know, text limit, but all the other days will be much longer and more detailed) **#fighting**

#stayingpositive #conversiondisorder #21DayPositivityChallenge
***

Picture: An overexposed selfie in front of a dark green brick wall, at [Redacted] Highschool. Taken on one of the days I actually made it to school. I have thick black winged eyeliner and bright red lipstick- a classic. **Oct 30, 2014.**

Caption: Day 2: "Crying doesn't indicate that you're weak. Since birth, it has always been a sign that you're alive." Today was more or less good, minus the fact that today felt so much like it was Friday- and the fact that I'm feeling really, really nostalgic. I'm glad that October is almost over- everything about Halloween depresses me. Simply the fact that I can't go trick or treating is upsetting, but also the memory of last Halloween; I tried going with my dad and my little brother, I probably lasted about 30 minutes before I just collapsed in the middle of the sidewalk crying, because I simply could not walk.

Soon after in November, I was diagnosed with conversion disorder. I'm going to do my best to stay positive tomorrow, enjoy myself, maybe even pass out candy for a bit. But if I feel anything like I do right now, I'll probably end up spending the evening in bed crying or sleeping the night away.

Also, [Redacted] (the bae) was talking about her schools Halloween dance, and said its probably better at home than it would be there, and it reminded me of the last dance I went to: It was the farewell dance for the eight graders, but all grades could attend- I was in seventh. All of my older friends were leaving literally the next day, the last day of school. So I danced with them the entire time, and I didn't even care how dumb I looked- I just danced, and I had such an amazing time. I want to dance like that, like nobody is around; I hate all these memories.

I'm considering going to the pep rally next week, especially since it's the last one for the year, but I have no idea how I could. It's supposed to be crowded as hell, from what I've heard. Pretty soon I'm going to, likely, arrange to do four periods a day. Not only will this be my second attempt, but we'll have to switch around my classes so that I can try to work in all my AP courses.

This scares me a little, because I hate change, especially in my every day routine, but I'm willing to keep my mind open. I am continuing to remind myself

"I /can/ walk" and that I /can/ do these things. My brain just isn't used to all this positivity. How sad-
#tobecontinued #21DayPositivityChallenge
*****

Picture: I'm smiling and holding a grape airhead candy over my mouth, and (yet again) my winged eyeliner is in-tact but partially cried off. **November 1st, 2014.**

Caption: Day three: (sorry this ones late, I was really tired last night!) "Sometimes you gotta fall before you fly, we're gonna work it out" Yesterday was, surprisingly, kind of amazing □ it started in the morning, and I was pretty upset about everything. My friends could tell I wasn't in a good mood. Then, skipping to second period, I was on my way to third, and I fell. I tried to get up once and I heard my knee crack; I thought it was nothing so I tried again, and every time I put pressure on my knee, I wanted to cry.

I was kind of just sitting in the middle of the hallway until a really nice girl from my second period (I wish I knew her name) saw me and she went and got the teacher, who called the nurses downstairs, who brought me a wheelchair.

The entire time I was terrified; I thought I was going to have to go to the hospital. I thought my mom would be upset with me. All these thoughts were swarming through my head for nothing- the only concerning thing about my knee is that there was one spot where it seemed to poke out a little, but I could bend it and walk on it just fine. They said to keep an eye on it so we did, and it didn't get any worse.

My mom and I were eating leftover pizza and watching Doctor Who when I decided "You know what, it's Halloween- we're going to watch something scary" so we spent about ten minutes going through Netflix when we decided on Carrie, the new one; it was really good. Not necessarily scary, but I liked it! Then we got about 40 minutes into Silence Of The Lambs when I got bored.

We put both of our jackolanterns outside (I'll post a picture in a bit) and our first trick-or-treater just so happened to be my brothers, friends, little sister- she recently turned four, and she's absolutely adorable c: Getting to see her was really nice, we talked to her mom for a bit. Sitting outside was really awful because the mosquitos were all over me-

My little brother went trick-or-treating for about and hour and gave me this airhead xD then, my older brother finally showed up; he's visiting from college, and it's really nice to see him. **#tobecontinued #21DayPositivityChallenge #candy #halloween #happy**

***

Picture: I think this is a photo I first saw on Tumblr, so it's not my original content. There's grey, cracked concrete with pretty purple flowers growing out of the crevices. I posted this for the symbolism behind it, I'm sure. **Nov 7th, 2014.**

Caption: I'm not dead! I'm so sorry I haven't been updating these past few days, I'm grounded until the end of the month ☐ but I can have wifi on the weekends, which is good. As for the 21 day positivity thing, I'm just going to have to start over. Today we had a follow up meeting about homebound, and it's been arranged that I'll be at school six out of seven periods a day; I'll even be going to lunch c: I want to be excited. I do. But I've fallen three times today, twice trying to stand up. I fell trying to get out of the shower and I just sat there for a good ten minutes crying because I simply /could not/ stand. When I walked out of the bathroom my dad asked if I was okay, and I said "No".

Then he asked if I was in pain, and again, I told him no. But I should've said yes. Have you ever done a lot of running or walked a really long distance to a point where your knees feel so weak you can hardly stand? Whenever I try to stand up my knees burn and feel weak. I have to, literally, lift all of my body weight with my arms. At the end of the day my arms feel bruised from using my walker all day. I broke. I did, what I consider, relapsing.. I looked up how to cure conversion disorder and everything they mentioned I've already done. I've done physical therapy. I go to counseling. I am now trialing my third anti-depressant. But the only way to cure conversion disorder is to learn how to cope with the cause, and to do that you need to find the trigger.. I have no idea what's triggered it.

The only reason I'm depressed is because of the conversion disorder. So I started googling diseases that cause paralysis..

I know for a fact that there's nothing wrong. All signs point to conversion disorder. But yet every time the phone rings a stupid part of me hopes that it's the doctor calling to say "We've figured it out; we need you to come here right away." Im in such denial about it. I hate that there's no exact cure for me; there's no medicine I can take, no surgery I could get. You just can't cure a mystery. Im constantly at war with my own mind and it's tearing me apart. This is not how I should be living my life. I just want to be normal again. **#conversiondisorder #fighting #sad**

 ***

Picture: It is a drawing, pretty nonsensical, but interesting to look at nonetheless. I used to pick quotes and then draw a bunch of random things around the words to make an overall picture; the quote here was "No one else deals with your demons, meaning that, maybe, defeating them could be the beginning of your meaning, friend." Not gonna lie...Twenty one Pilots still holds up for me. **Dec 30th, 2014.**

Caption: "No one else deals with your demons; Meaning that maybe defeating them could be the beginning of your meaning, friend." Twenty One Pilots, Kitchen sink

I hate being the way I am- I'm significantly insignificant. Everywhere I go, the moment I walk into a room, people notice me. They hear me coming, the sound of plastic touching the floor and metal shifting, then I stop every few steps to take a break; Old people stare at me. Babies and small animals don't like to come near me because the sound of my walker scares them.

Not only do I get unwanted attention, but unnecessary help. I can't stand up and take two steps without people rushing to my side, insisting that I sit back down and that they'll do whatever I was about to do for me.

If I fall, people act like I need an ambulance, when really all I need is a chair to help me up. I get asked the question all the time "Does it hurt?" for some reason, and yeah, it does, in lots of different ways; the constant back pain, soreness of my arms, the shaking/weakness in the knees, the chalices all over my hands. I want nothing more than to be insignificant, unnoticed. Just in a different way than I already am.

I'm beginning to get tired of telling people that they will "never be alone in this world" when there's seldom a time I don't feel isolated. I have a rare disorder that not many people, even most doctors, know about. Being insignificant is always going to be impossible with my walker. But if everyone is going to notice me, I want them to notice /more/ than just my walker. I want them to notice I have a health condition, "It's called conversion disorder" I'll tell them, and I want them to acknowledge that and put effort into understanding and caring about it. Nobody pays attention to what's actually wrong with me. My disorder is rare and unknown, making it unimportant to the world even though this is who /I/ am.

They'll help me up, walk me to class, ask me if I'm in pain. But if I tell them why, tell them what's actually wrong, they don't care. It's too complex for them to understand, so they brush it off, and I remain unknown. **#tbc #continuedincomments #rant #sorry #insignificant**

(Then, in the comments I finish with):

I just want to be known. I want to spread the awareness of conversion disorder so that it's NOT some random thing no one knows about. I want to try to enhance the understanding of it to my teachers, doctors, and peers. But nobody actually cares to listen, because I'm just a daisy in a field of sunflowers. I'm insignificant. And I can't stand it.

***

Picture: It's showing half of a grandfather clock that's antique and pretty to look at, though I'm pretty sure I took this picture at a funeral home. A little weird. **Jan 1st, 2016.**

Caption:

I feel like I'm a fuckboy, and 2016 is a nice girl Ijust started dating six hours ago. "Haha, soooo, what now? ;) am I going to learn to walk again? Will I find out what's wrong with me? Am I going to get in a relationship? Will I get any new pets? What about school, how will my grades be? ;)))" and when 2016 shyly replies "Well, let's see what time has in store for us!" I just get pissy and already disinterested.

"Who cares about 'New Years resolutions' or any of that "New year, new me" bullshit. It's January again, so fucking what?" And, in this metaphorical insecure girl+horny impatient fuckboy equation, 2016 might do something just to keep me happy, like, in an instant I could magically walk again. But that's just not how things work.

Time isn't something you can bend to your will, no matter how much you actually try, because trying to rush positive lifestyles is just a big fat waste of time. **#rant #thoughts #newyear #2016**
***

<u>YouTube Archive</u>

When I realized that there was no hope in fighting my diagnosis of Conversion Disorder, I decided to dive into my "healing journey" head-on and create a YouTube channel to document everything on video. I introduced myself with a video explaining what Conversion Disorder is and how it affected me, personally. I have had these videos privated for many years now because it was very triggering to be reminded of the self-imposed brainwashing I underwent as a means of survival; I was not allowed to fight for myself, so I did my best to accept a diagnosis I knew was wrong.

I have typed out a complete transcription of each video, and they are all public to watch on **my YouTube channel under the name "Ivy Babbitt".** You can read along while watching the videos if you would like to have an additional visual aspect to keep in mind as you read my story. *(Skip to page 69 for the beginning of the story)*

Title: I Have Conversion Disorder
Posted on **January 3rd, 2015**

Transcription:

Hi. My name is Ivy, I'm 14 years old, and I have "Conversion Disorder." You might not know what that means, and that's okay, because the reason I started this channel was to spread awareness about my disorder and help others while helping myself. Conversion disorder is a condition in which mental symptoms – stress, anxiety, depression, etc. – show in physical ways. It can take form in many ways: seizures, blindness, losing the ability to walk, talk.

My case of Conversion Disorder converts stress and social anxiety into paralysis, making it very difficult to walk. I use a walker to get around, and I try to exercise my legs daily. [shows my walker to the camera] See? This is a horrible view. It started showing around the time I began sixth grade, and ever since then, it's been slowly progressing. I wasn't diagnosed until halfway through my seventh-grade year, and it still took over a year and a half to come to terms with it.

I'm now starting the second semester of my freshman year. Today's date is January 2nd, 2015, meaning that we are two days into the new year. I'm gonna share with you guys three of my New Year's resolutions: one, make a YouTube channel so I can make vlogs documenting my recovery. Two, a year from now, I'd like to be able to walk completely unassisted. And three, spread the awareness of Conversion Disorder.

I'm tired of being unnoticed. Now, hear me out; I mean this in the least conceited way possible! I have a rare condition that not many people, including doctors, know about. All the attention I get is because I have a walker. The moment I walk into the room, the first thing anyone notices about me is, "Hey, that person is disabled," and everyone's really kind about it, too. I mean, like, they'll urge me to sit back down so I don't have to do any extra work, and if I fall, it's like a race to get there to see who can help me up first.

People are always asking if I'm in pain. It's all really nice, but the moment I start to explain, "Oh, I have Conversion Disorder," I'll tell them, they stop caring. It's such a complex, unknown disease that people would rather brush it off than acknowledge its existence, and that really upsets me.

This time next year, I will be able to walk. This time next year, Conversion Disorder will no longer be a stigma that gets brushed under the rug the moment its name is said out loud, because I am going to make a

Youtube channel and post vlogs to give people a chance to see firsthand what it's like living with Conversion Disorder. Throughout this entire time I will be fighting towards overcoming this disease and I will walk down the school hallways without everyone being able to know that I am coming by the sound of my walker.

These three resolutions may sound small and unimportant, and Conversion Disorder may just sound like another sad story that you don't have time to listen to, but any and all empathy given to me because of my condition does NOT count unless you acknowledge my existence while doing so. I have Conversion Disorder. Every day is a battle where I go at war with my mind. I'm trying to gain the ability to control my own body. This is me; Conversion Disorder is a huge part of who I am, and by ignoring that, you're ignoring me, making me nothing but significant insignificance.

My name is Ivy, I have Conversion Disorder, and I'd like to tell you my story. It would mean the world to me if you would listen.

Title: Video Diary #1; Homeschooling
Posted on **January 12th, 2015**

Description: My first video diary documenting my recovery with conversion disorder :) I mostly made this for my own purposes, but as always, I'd like to make it available to anyone else who may receive any kind of help from it. I feel like I made some major accomplishments today, I'm proud! Hopefully a good start will lead to a good end.

Transcription:

[sighs, covers face] Hi, everyone. Basically, I've been procrastinating making any videos and… I don't know, I might not even post this. I just think that it would be good to use my channel for its intended purpose. I'm going to count this as, I guess, a video diary? Um, I don't know if I'm going to do an ongoing video diary. It might be nice! I mean, I don't know, let's see how this goes. Today's date is January 12th, 2015, and I got four hours of sleep last night. Yay.

I'm so done, and I'm scared; today is the…well, not necessarily the "first" *[air quotes]* day…I haven't been to school since last Tuesday, so there's going to be three days plus today's work, because I'm not going today, because today is the first day I'm starting home schooling? I mean, basically…yeah, it's homeschooling, because I'm not going to be going to school at all.

First it was three classes a day, and then we made it four, and then we made it six and my mom decided that, no, I just couldn't go to school at all if I was going to focus at all on re-learning to walk. So I'm going to be a full-time homeschooling student, and that thought terrifies me! I can just imagine all my work, like, piling up and then having to drop out of all my AP classes; I'm in all advanced classes, minus geography, because I got behind in that class.

I don't know, I just… like, three fourths of last night was just me staying up freaking out, going "oh my god, I'm gonna fail. I'm not gonna get to go to college, I'm gonna get held back, and I'm not going to be able to, like…get a good job. I want to help people in the future. Oh my god!" and it's just…*[shakes head, sighs]*.

If anyone out there watching also does homeschool, it would be so amazing to hear about your experiences with it. You know, how you manage it, if it's efficient.

I'm just clueless right now. It's really hard because I'm going through so many things that not a lot of people know how to relate to. Like, I don't know, I'll stay up all night trying to help someone and trying to relate to their situation, even though the moment I meet someone going through something even relatively similar to what I am, I just break down in tears. I'm like, what? You have Conversion Disorder? Or, what? You're homeschooled, too? It…it's sad.

It's not all sad though, really! Like, I can already tell my legs are getting kind of stronger? I mean, I'm trying to stay positive about it, even though it scares me whenever things are getting good, because…recovery, as much as people would like to believe that it's like this *[motions a straight, upward line]* it's like that *[motions a wavy, inconsistent path]*.

I'm going to attempt to show you guys my walking, if I can figure out how to technology. I'm recording with my iPod with a free app I got on the download store, and I don't know what I'm doing. Basically, I'm going to set you on the ground and hope you can see what I'm doing. This is very complicated, I'm making this way harder than it needs to be. Oh my gosh, I'm sorry about my pale vampire feet, if you can even see them. *[shuffles about 10 feet away to stand in view of the camera]*

But basically, what I've been doing to practice walking is: I put my walker in front of me, like so, and I just walk towards it *[takes a few steps forward]* oh my god, I'm doing amazing! This is amazing. [knees buckling, I grab onto the walker] I am not falling, because this is not the time for falling. Oh guys, I'm so happy!

I am going to attempt to do one more scene like that, if I can, which I think I can. I'm really excited about today. My legs are like, extremely…working, you know? [takes anothers few steps towards the walker] like, look at that! Oh my god, I could run. I'm just like… *[quickly walks in the other direction, then leans onto something out of view while catching my breath]* walking. Wait, let me stop it *[pauses recording, sits back down]*.

I know it seems really stupid to get excited over walking two feet, but that's honestly a major achievement for me, and I don't know, I'm gonna let myself be proud, because this is amazing.

I mean, it's good! I'm sorry if this is boring. I don't know, I think I'm going to upload this, but for my purposes, and maybe in the future it will help other people. That would just make it all the more better.

Basically, I am just really happy with how this came out. Last night was really awful, I stayed up super late because I absolutely could not sleep, and no matter what I did I was just panicking, and oh my gosh, overthinking, and it was awful. Now I actually feel really great, and I don't know, any and all support from you guys absolutely means the world to me. I'm just so glad to have some way of sharing my story with everyone, I don't know.

One view or one hundred views, or a thousand views, I don't care how many! As long as I know that there are people out there listening and that there are people that care, it honestly means the world to me. I hope everyone had or is having a wonderful Monday, and my mom is home, so I'm gonna go. I love you all, you are beautiful, amazing, stay awesome.

Title: Video Diary #2; Old people
Posted on **January 18th, 2015**

Description:
This one was actually filmed on Thursday (1/15/15) but I was having trouble finding time to upload it (procrastinating and sleeping all day) It's been a little rough these past few days. I'll definitely be updating later this afternoon. Thank you for watching :)

Transcription:

Hey, everyone! I spent the last 10 minutes trying to set my iPod up so I wouldn't have to hold it while I'm recording, and…*[screen slowly points toward the ceiling]* so, that's all fun. By the way, if I kind of look like I just woke up from a five hour nap, I did, because today was eventfully uneventful for me. I actually left the house and went to two places which is highly traumatic for my mind and my body, but I think I did pretty well. Literally all we did was we went to the doctors office to pick up paperwork, and then we went to Office Depot to make copies of the paperwork. I got to walk around to look at pens while my mom made copies, so yeah, really wild.

I haven't made a video since Monday because, like, today I have absolutely nothing to talk about. But you know, the show must go on, so I'm going to make myself look like a loser in front of a camera! Just kidding. I'll talk for about four minutes and count that as one of my daily video diaries. I don't think it's gonna be a daily thing. I mean, maybe? But I feel like I should talk about today.

Umm, okay. So the fact that I have…"social anxiety" *[puts my head down]* alright, I have social anxiety, and I try to deny it. Like, I always go around and I'm just like "I don't care what people think about me, I'm awesome!" But honestly, I care a lot. I mean, today I actually counted the amount of old people who gave me sad stares, and it was seven. Whenever I go out places, everyone– little kids, old people, people my age– they all stare at me, and they're just like, "oh my gosh, a walker? I might have one of those someday" and it's like…it makes me really upset.

Me and my mom had a whole conversation with a nice lady from the doctor's office about the little shoes at the bottom of my walker. Actually, I think I'll show them. I think they're really adorable. *[shows a view of my walker, gesturing towards the floor]*

Okay, if anyone was wondering, they're called "walker gliders" and I got mine online at Walmart, but you can probably find them tons of other places. All you have to do is google it. They serve the same purpose as when people put tennis balls on the ends of their walker, but they kind of give my walker way more personality, and it's a conversational topic.

But yeah, it just really sucks being noticed because of it. A little baby boy had to be dragged out of the room by his mother because he wanted to touch and look at my walker, and she was like "come on, we gotta go". I was like "oh my god, I'm so sorry!" But um, it was okay. I mean, I'm pretty good, I think the whole *"going out places"* really tired me out considering I've been asleep since 11:30 and it's now 3:00

One other place that we went to was a restaurant for breakfast called "Andy's Kitchen". Apparently it's been around since my mom was like, five, so it's been around for a while. I'm not calling you old, mom, I swear! That was really nice, there were a lot of really nice people there. Of course, more people stared, but you know, I don't care…I mean, I do care, but oh well. I thought I would also update on my legs; I don't know, I wanted to update you guys on how much stronger my legs are getting, and it's actually amazing. We spent about 20 minutes last night just walking in the living room and every two steps my mom had to stop me because she was freaking out and hugging me, like, "Ivy, I'm so proud!" and I was like…*[laughs uncomfortably]*

Last week I could barely pick up either of my legs from a sitting position, and now I can do this! *[shows myself in a seated position, bending my leg at the knee to elevate it]* oh, look at that! Wow, so good! Oh, look at that, that's amazing. Wow! Like, I can lift my feet like…five inches off the ground. I'm so proud. I've also been doing like, I guess, marching things? That's what my mom calls it, where I kind of just stand in place and lift my feet *[shows myself standing up and doing a marching-type exercise]* Look at that, oh my gosh. But yeah, you guys like my socks? Because I like my socks. Um, okay, I think I'm going to bring this to an end.

I just wanted to say thank you so much for spending the time to watch this and follow my story. I actually got my first comment on the video yesterday…on the one about me having conversion disorder, and it was by Tacy Thompson? I really hope I'm saying it right. So, a shout out to you for knowing what Conversion Disorder is, you honestly made my week. Shout out to everyone else who is watching. You know, every little bit of support counts and really helps me just go that extra mile every day. Even just your view on this video is going to give me so much hope, and it really just means so much to me. Before this gets all sentimental, I'm gonna say goodbye, because I don't want to cry in front of you guys.

I hope you guys all are having an amazing day/afternoon/morning, wherever you are…um, I just wanted to take a minute to say: I'm so proud of making it through another week. Like, look at you, you're so amazing!

You should really count it as an accomplishment… I'm so proud of you. You have been so strong and you're only going to keep getting stronger. Honestly, the fact that you're watching this right now makes you one of my many, many inspirations, because just getting out of bed in the morning and doing stuff…that's a lot…you are perfect, and you should never let anyone tell you anything less. So yeah, I hope everyone enjoyed this; I don't know if it's enjoyable, I'm pretty boring. But yeah, um, thank you for watching.

Title: Video Diary #3; School again?
Posted on January 20th, 2015

Description:
Link to my tumblr; **http://keep-moving--forward--x.tumblr.com/**

As promised in the video, I will let you read (optional) what I wrote today, and why I'm not doing very well right now. It's a bit lengthy, and if you are easily triggered by text including mentions of suicide, depression, ect. (Also, there is mild cussing) I strongly urge you to not scroll down. The last thing I would want from posting this is for it to have a harmful effect on someone else; sorry it's so long, and highly pessimistic. Thank you for taking the time to watch my videos and sit through all my rambling. You truly are what's going to keep me going at the end of the day. Thank you.
***

Sitting. Sitting here on a stupid toilet, head propped up by my hand, staring at the ugly yellow tiles that are becoming burned into my memory. My legs are already tingling and falling deeply asleep at an alarming yet expected rate, and I want nothing more than to just fall with them. Im not tired. I went to bed at a reasonable time last night, had a cup of coffee this morning. Im simply exhausted. I don't see the point of getting out of bed in the morning if by the third period of the day, my favorite class, I'll just be sitting in a dirty bathroom stall crying, hyperventilating, and numb. I don't even know what's worse anymore; feeling nothing, or feeling everything. I literally think I'm right in the middle of the two, if such a place even exists.

One part of me wants to cry, scream at the top of my lungs about how unfair everything is until my vocal cords are ripped to shreds, because it's not, it's not fair! I want to live my life, pursue my greatest aspirations. Change the world. Get straight A's, go to college, get married, have kids- I have so much damn potential. And all that potential is going straight down the drain, with every stumble, trip, fall, crash; it's all for naught. I'm only getting older, only coming closer to dying, and a part of me is infuriated by this; while the other part can't help but be glad. This disease is debilitating. Every day is a battle where I go at war with my own mind trying to gain the ability to control my own body. I've spent the last four years fighting. From the moment I wake up to the moment I go back to bed is a struggle- everything is a struggle. I stare at random people doing random things like bending down to pick something up without falling, or standing up out of a chair without using their arms to lift them up in utter amazement. I can't go hang out at the mall. I can't walk around, I probably won't be able to drive in a year in a half when I turn sixteen, shit, I can't even take a fucking shower without a god damn chair to sit in.

My entire existence is miserable. Im in highschool and I have a fucking walker. Talk about a self confidence boost, am I right? I keep my eyes on the ground at all times and try to pretend I don't know people stare, I always wait until I'm home and alone before I cry. Part of me wants to live.

I want to fight and overcome this godforsaken disorder so bad- but it's so hard, that the other part of me wants nothing more than to just not have to do it anymore. I want to lay in bed at all times from the moment the sun rises to the very second the sun sets, just to sleep the day away. Then stay up all night feeling sorry for myself, having random bursts of determination to actually do something, which never lead anywhere. Part of me would rather die than survive, because that's all I'm really doing anymore.

Lately it seems as though I'm constantly on the brink of suicide, even though I'll spend countless hours telling others that it's "never the answer" and that its "a permanent solution to a temporary problem" and all that jazz, and this really worries me. I don't want to die. But at the same time, I definitely don't want to live if this is all life has in store for me. Part of me is freaking out over the fact that I just skipped class; am I going to get in trouble? What if the school calls, what will I tell mom? Though the other part doesn't really give two shits about what happens anymore.

***

Transcription:

[sighs] Hi, guys. This video is not going to be as upbeat and happy as the last ones, but, as you can tell: I figured out a way to set my iPod so I can record hands free! So, that's pretty cool. Today was not fun, um [pause] so, update… I'm not really homeschooled, apparently. Well…yeah, I don't know if I was homeschooled before, but I'm definitely not now. It was going to be, you know, I stay home all day every day, but my mom eventually came to the conclusion (after all the crap the school system is giving us) that I do need to be at school every day. So, I'm back to doing three periods a day, this being my first day back.

I don't know if it's that, or if it's the fact that today was when they decided to give everyone their new semester schedules– even though nothing changed on my schedule so there's still so much extra walking– but, I don't know, today was really horrible. Um, I don't even want to get into it in this video; if you want to read about why, you can read about it in the description. It's kind of a thing I wrote during third period.

I wish I had something happier to talk about. I mean, something cool is that I made a new Tumblr, and I kind of got as far as trying to make my tumblr look attractive and nice and *[jazz hands]* wow…and I spent about three hours, then I was like, forget this. It looks pretty cool now, so I will definitely put the link to that in the description!

I'm really planning on being very active on it. I want it to go with my Youtube channel, but kind of like a personal account, because I've always wanted one of those really pretty Tumblr's where all you post is black and white, and you only post pictures of trees and water…I just can't do that. So, I think it's going to be more of a writing account, maybe with occasional pictures, who knows? I don't know, I just know that I'm going to be writing a lot and posting a lot of writing on there, so I will definitely be posting on my Tumblr what I will be posting in the description [of this video].

Um, my walking's getting worse. I mean, it's to be expected, it's not a bad type of "getting worse", but it's not getting better at the moment. I'm very worried about a new weird symptom type thingy that I've noticed…my right leg has started shaking really bad, like, a lot; most times it's when I stand up, and it's kind of scary, actually. I think the reason why it worries me so much is because most people you see with Conversion Disorder have seizures and tremors and they can't talk, and I'm nowhere near that bad! I don't want to get that bad, you know? I told my mom and she said it's probably just muscle spasms because I'm actually using my legs, and I mean, I guess that's a reasonable explanation. I don't know. So I'm trying not to worry about that so I'm not piling a bunch of stress on me, because…*[shrugs]* that's not good for me.

I want to know how YOU guys are doing. I mean, I know, like, probably 10 people watch my videos, but something that you should know about me is that I really love whenever people who read or watch my stuff comment below and tell me how they're doing, because I just love talking to people and hearing all their stories. It just makes me so happy. So, tell me if you are having a good week so far, what you did for

Martin Luther King Jr. Day; if you stayed home or went to school. I stayed home.

Um, this video is very unorganized and very not good but, um, yeah. I thought it'd be nice to update. *[continues in different room]* By the way, I'm sorry about the random room change, um, my mom got home. I wanted to end this video properly, so, that's it, basically. Um, I will keep you updated as frequently as possible. Tomorrow I'm going to start seeing a new psychologist, and I'm pretty sure I've met her before, so I'm pretty excited about it. My old one wasn't as qualified as this one, I guess you could say, and I don't know, I'm really excited. I will definitely, definitely, definitely– this is a pinky promise, I promise I won't break this one– I will definitely tell you how it went tomorrow sometime, or the day after tomorrow, but no later than that.

So yeah, um, thank you so much for watching this and I really hope you're doing well. If you're not, then you should totally leave me a comment or a message. So yeah, you are amazing, and thank you so much!

Title: Video Diary #4;
Posted on January 21st, 2015

Description:

This Video pretty much speaks for itself; my mind is weirdly blank at the moment- Follow me on tumblr, maybe? **https://www.tumblr.com/blog/keep-moving--forward---x** Thank you so much for taking the time to watch this, and, just a reminder, you're amazing. Don't forget that.

Transcription:

Hello, everyone. I think I would like to start this video by saying that yesterday was not a good day; it was one of those days where I kind of just had a mental breakdown, and everything was like, piling, and it was like, ugh. But I'm a lot better now! Actually, today I feel really great. I mean, I put on real clothes and I did my hair, and I'm actually wearing my glasses. I promised I would tell you guys about how it went with my new psychologist; well, she's not actually a psychologist, as I found out. It's not like I expected it was going to be.

When we had gotten to her office there was this cactus with a spider web on it, and I thought it was the prettiest thing ever. I took a picture of it and then I got into a weird mood where you're just inspired by everything, so I took a bunch of pictures, and I'm definitely going to post them on my Tumblr so you guys can look at that. So, okay…we get there and she's not who I thought it was going to be. I thought I knew her, but I didn't. Just after the first session I can tell that she's very professional and she's had so much experience. She actually counseled my first psychiatrist, and I think that's kind of amazing!

So far we haven't really done a lot of the "therapy stuff" because it was just the first session. My mom was there the whole time and we kind of got more of a background, so she's like, how are you doing in school? What's the problem here? I am already in love, though, because when I brought up Conversion Disorder she knew exactly what I was talking about, and I was like "wait, are you sure?" She's really nice and she's super professional, extremely professional, and I'm honestly really looking forward to not only working with her, but, you know, seeing her.

This video is very unorganized…speaking of organization: Okay, I have a new plan type thing for videos… I really do like doing the video diaries and I kind of like these being an improvised thing, but I'm going to start making actual videos about actual things and whatnot. Obviously, as you probably can tell, I'm horrible at giving oral presentations that are improvised. I'm super awkward, and I'm just like…yeah, awkward head movements. So my new plan is that I'm going to actually use some of the stuff I've written, but whenever I write journals I'm going to actually make them into videos and say the things out loud. I mean, it's kind of like having a script, so it's not as intimidating…but yeah, um, that's something that I think I'm really going to try to start as soon as possible.

I would like to say that I feel really bad for being so negative lately, so I figured I would give you guys an update on my legs and my walking. Actually, I have a cane too, it matches my walker, look [shows my blue cane] isn't that adorable?

I actually eventually came to the conclusion that I don't know how to use it, so I did look up a YouTube video about how to properly walk with a cane, and it all sounds really stupid…but it's actually kind of complicated. I'm just like, wait, what am I doing with my legs, and how do I do this? I'm really gonna need to work towards using my cane. For now, it's unsafe to use it at all times, I really do need to stick with my walker for now.

But I do like practicing with it because it's actually kind of fun after a while, once you actually, like, know what you're doing! So, I thought I could show you guys…*[shows myself walking towards the camera with my cane]* Oh, okay, I don't think this is the best view…but I basically…okay, I'm going to use the chair, because gravity *[grabs onto desk chair]*.

Um, basically, the way the videos described it is: you put your cane first, and you put your bad foot first… so I put my left foot first, because that's the weaker one, and…look at that! This makes me so happy, like, this is amazing. Oh my god, I might actually be able to do this really soon…

So basically, that's all I really have for today. Thank you so much for watching this. I don't know, it's just so weird how one day I'm just like, I don't even want to..I don't know. Definitely some videos you can be on the lookout for: I really, really want to post an entire video about alternatives and coping skills to self-harm and things like that, because I know that it's been getting kind of bad for me lately in that general area, and I know that so many people [struggle].

I mean, it really is debilitating, and I will be the first one to tell you that no matter how bad it hurts when you're crying so hard that you can barely breathe at night, it's going to feel so much better in the morning when you wake up and you see your dog. Or, you find a flower and you pick it because it's really pretty, or you take a really nice selfie!

It's just so weird how the littlest things can kind of just make the world of a difference. Does that make any sense? So I absolutely will be making a video on that, and, I don't know, I have a lot of plans. I'm pretty excited to see how they work out…yeah, this is getting long and I'm getting weird because I'm very tired, so I'm gonna take a nap, probably.

It's already Wednesday, wow, the middle of the week! You've made it this far, and you are so close to Friday, and I'm so proud of you. I just want everyone to know that no matter how horrible it seems right now, it's going to get better. I'm trying to think of the least cliche way possible to say this, but, at my school they have a quote wall in one of the English hallways…I walk past it everyday, and honestly, a lot of those quotes have really kept me going. One of my favorite quotes on there is: "It's just a bad day, not a bad life". It's true! There's so many quotes and I actually also want to make a list of them for people to look at.

Have you ever seen those posts where they're just like, you know, "a year ago I was broke, jobless, homeless… and now I just got the key to my first house"? Theres the one where she says that when she was 18 she was depressed and suicidal, and now she's sitting on the couch and she can hear her husband in the other room reading her children a bedtime story, and…I don't know, I just think things like that are really inspiring, and not in a stupid way…you can see that it really does get better…

I'm gonna go before I waste any more of your time…you're amazing, I love you, I'm so proud of you. Thank you for watching, it means everything to me.

Title: Video Diary #5; Too tired to think of a title
Posted on January 22nd, 2015

Description:
Or a description. Follow me on tumblr!

Transcription:

Hi! Okay, um, I'm going to keep this vlog short and sweet to the point, and then I'm gonna go back to bed…I didn't go to school yesterday because of my appointment…I was supposed to go to school today, so I got ready– I got dressed, I didn't really do my hair because I'm lazy– I put on shoes, and I did all that good stuff. I was feeling really weak, and…I mean, I always feel weak in the morning; It's kind of just something I've gotten used to. But lately it's been getting worse, so I even wrote myself a little note: *[shows handwritten note that says "You can do this. You're strong. And you look really cute today."]* and I posted it on my Tumblr, which you guys should go follow, if you want, maybe?

I was just like, you know what, I can do this! So got up and I went to brush my teeth, and I fell. Then I got up and on the way to the living room I almost fell again, and my mom just…she can hear from the other room every time I fall. She always immediately asks "Are you okay?" and I'm always okay. She asked, "Can you get up?", and most the time, yes, I can get up. But she was just like, "Ivy, I think you need to stay home, can you go today?" and I said, "I'm gonna try", which was my way of saying "No, but I'm gonna do it anyways"…

The main thing I wanted to talk about in this vlog, though…because this is a huge issue that not a lot of adults are willing to acknowledge, and it's getting to a point where it's taking such a huge toll on my health that I don't want to get out of bed in the morning anymore…the school systems today value education more than they value health for each student that goes to school. They get money, and if you miss more than 10 days a year, they don't get paid for you, which is why you're not allowed to miss more than that. They'll sue you if you do! So, I'm here and I can't really walk out of the house, so how am I supposed to walk around school all day and do a full schedule?

At my last 504 meeting the lady told my mom, like, "Oh, well, we'll just get Ivy a wheelchair and we will have someone wheel her around so she can be here all day". My mom was like "The hell you will!" I don't want to be in a wheelchair, and I know my mom doesn't want it, and I know my doctors don't want it…putting me in a wheelchair would give me a sense of hopelessness, like, "okay, this is it, I'm just not gonna walk and I'm just gonna be stuck in a wheelchair for the rest of my life".

Our main goal is for me to be granted the ability to stay home and do schooling from home until I can walk again. I can't focus on my walking at school because I'm not really focusing on how well I'm walking, I'm focusing on [getting to class] before the bell rings so I'm not caught in the middle of traffic. That alone is very stressful, but then adding on top of that, I am almost 15, and I'm in highschool while having to walk with a walker. I don't think the teachers understand how frustrating that is. You know, for the longest time I've always had this attitude where I'm just like, you know what, I don't wake up to impress you every day! I'm awesome, I'm amazing, I can do whatever I want! I can look however I want, I can act however I want, and it doesn't matter what you think, because I love myself. But lately it's gotten to the point where I don't think like that anymore…having a walker has made me doubt myself and doubt my abilities, you know?

I've been in a mood lately where I'm just kind of like, "no one's ever gonna like me, I'm not gonna be able to get married someday, I'm never gonna be able to walk"…it's just a bunch of horrible negative crap and it really takes a toll on my self-esteem. I hate being that girl with the walker, and if they would just give me time off from school and allow me to stay home until I can walk again, I could go back to school perfectly fine by the last nine weeks. I could probably be walking without anything, or just with a cane, and that alone would just be huge…so yeah, be on the lookout for that video coming soon. It's my main priority right now.

Um, my next video I post will either be a video diary or a whole video about how the school's education system values education more than they value health. I realize I'm rambling and I'm starting to stutter, which is weird, so I'm gonna go. I'm really sorry about this; I wanted to have, like, a positivity streak…but I guess that's not happening. Uh, it's Thursday, tomorrow is Friday! Oh my god, you've made it almost through an entire week, wow. I'm really proud of you, and you should be proud of yourself, too.

I know I say this in the end of like, every video, but I really hope that you understand how amazing it is that you got out of bed this morning. You may or may not have gone to school, but even if you didn't, you did stuff; you put clothes on and you brushed your teeth, and little things like that are amazing.

Ever since I was little, all these teachers would tell me "don't make a mountain out of a molehill", because I would always over-exaggerate and make things so much harder than they needed to be. Now I always have to remind myself that you shouldn't make a molehill out of a mountain! Like, you walked three steps without your walker? Oh my god, huge accomplishment. You got out of bed this morning? Oh my god, you deserve a freaking award, because you are awesome…never let anyone else make you doubt yourself, because you, my friend, are true perfection…and that's all there is to it!

So yeah, thank you for watching, I will keep you updated and post again as soon as possible. I'm going to try to be a little active on my Tumblr today, maybe? Maybe not. Yeah, thank you so much, you're amazing. Thank you for your support.

Title: Video Diary 6; What Not to do in the ER
Posted on January 27th, 2015

Description:

People these days need to realize that the
///emergency/// room is for ///emergencies/// I hope you
enjoyed this! Follow me on tumblr, maybe?
http://sighvy.tumblr.com/ (my new url is "sighvy")
(idk i kinda love it) My kik is *[redacted]* Thank you :)

Transcription:
Hi, guys! Since I posted my last video it's gotten
about 12 views, which isn't a lot, but it's something, so
that's really cool. I'm actually making this video more
as an update for anyone who wants to watch, and for
documentation purposes, so please forgive me. My
iPod is not working with me today and I don't have the
patience to fix it…

I have a really bad headache– I've had it since
yesterday– and I will tell you why…my mom had a lot
of errands to run yesterday, and halfway through the

amount of time she was gone, I fell…falling, ever since July [last year] has been a very scary experience for me, because back in the summer I fell and I broke my pinky toe. It wasn't just like, oh whatever, just tape it together…it was like, oh my god, her bone sticking out, type thing. So I dropped my iPod and I went to pick it up, and I fell. I got really scared and I touched my toe, and I was like, "okay, it's not broken"…a few minutes later I looked down and I was like, "oh I'm bleeding!" So I went to the bathroom and I was like "this is gross", and then as I was cleaning it, I went to see what was wrong with it because it started hurting…where they stitched it back in July, after I had surgery, was ripped; that's the point where I started freaking out.

So I was going to wait for my mom and dad to come home, and my friend was like, "You've got to call her now". So I was like, "okay fine" and it was terrifying because I was so scared, and it ended up being just a completely stupid, like, whatever. Mom was actually, like, overly calm about it. She was like "okay, let's go get some x-rays, but can we go to Mcdonald's first?" and I was like, "yeah okay, sure!". I wasn't in a lot of pain and it wasn't anything serious; it wasn't gushing blood, there was no bones.

So we went and got my dad and we went to Whataburger, and then we went to the ER. We get there and it is full of people. There are literally two chairs left, which is where my mom and my dad sit, and I was in a wheelchair. There are screaming children, runny-nosed babies, angry parents, and I was just like…this is gonna take a while. Within about three hours we started to get all impatient and we were like, okay, this is a little ridiculous…that's when my dad left so that he could go home and do a few things, and then he was gonna pick up my brother at four.
Around five is when we were like, "okay, why is everybody getting called in except us?" The thing is, by then the only people who had gotten there that were there BEFORE us were these two people, and they weren't getting called in either!

All these new people were getting called in, so we asked the nurse, like, what's going on? I'm in pain and I have an open wound– a possible broken toe– and all these other people are getting called in. There were screaming children who were running in circles, and there were stupid teenage girls walking out like flipping their hair and, like, rolling their eyes…I was like, I'm going to punch you in the face, because nothing's obviously wrong with you! I was sitting there, like, on the verge of tears because it was hurting really bad, and I was just like, "I need to see a doctor".

Given the fact that it's flu season, a bunch of people are going to go to the ER, and I get that, but if you're taking your kid to the ER because they're congested or their nose won't stop running? Take them to a doctor! I'm going to tell you guys something really cool…so, you know how they call it the ER? It actually stands for EMERGENCY room. Isn't that awesome? I mean, I knew that, but apparently a bunch of people don't…a lot of people were so concerned about their kid who was coughing that they were prioritized over a possible broken toe…the nurse literally said "ma'am, you have to wait your turn, we see our patient in order and order by severity".I have no idea how a runny nose is more severe than a possible broken toe, but I mean, whatever.

We demanded that we get X-Rays and we finally did. They took three pictures and there was only one picture where the tip looked kind of off, and my mom was like, "you know what? If it's broken, you can call us. We're going home", and they haven't called since. So uh, yeah, I don't know. It doesn't look broken. It still kind of hurts, but it doesn't feel broken, I can move it and it's not bleeding anymore…

One more thing: I did see my therapist today, and tomorrow I have an appointment with an actual psychologist for the very first time. I'm going to see a real psychologist, and I'm excited about that…it's just the evaluation meeting, which is always boring…I was gonna go to school tomorrow because I had my 504 meeting today, and everything is all worked out, and everything's perfect. I can go back to school and I'm really excited about that. I got my schedule made to my accommodations and uh, hopefully I can go back Thursday. If not, then, I don't know. Um, tell me how you guys are doing, if you're even watching this.

Um, yeah, I will continue to keep my Tumblr updated. I took a bunch of selfies today if anyone's interested in that. I tried changing my url and I thought everything got deleted, I was super scared for like two hours, and I was like "what did I do?". But now it's all back to normal. My new url is, um…I don't even like saying it out loud because it looks so funny, like, you're going to laugh whenever you read it, but if you say it out loud you're just like "what?". So, I'm gonna put the link to my Tumblr below, and you can look at it. You can follow me if you want, I follow most people back.

It's halfway through the week, you only got two more days till Friday! I'm so proud of you. You can totally do this, and I hope you're doing well, and if you're not you can leave me a comment (which I prefer you don't, because I will probably not even know how to reply, Youtube is super complicated…I think I have a notification right now that I haven't read)...but um, I'll actually leave my Kik below, too, for the matter of [messaging].

Thank you so so much for watching, and I hope the rest of your day/morning, or evening, goes well. I will keep you updated.

Title: Video Diary #7; Superbowl
Posted on February 1st, 2015

Description:

Follow me on tumblr, maybe? **http://sighvy.tumblr.com/** So, yeah. Today was rough, and I've spent the last 45 minutes trying to come up with a decent description for this video but I am too tired to write- hopefully, probably, tomorrow. I guess the video can speak for itself. I hope you enjoyed :)

Transcription:

Hello, everyone! First things first: let's take a moment to appreciate how adorable my outfit is, like, wow! I wore this necklace and my pants, but you can't see them…actually, you will see them, because towards the end at this video I think I'm going to give another leg update…I don't know if I've done one of those recently, I feel like it's been a while…this is, as you can already tell by the title, just a video diary. So it's basically an update. By the way, my hair is all windblown from being in the car, and my eyeliner is disgusting from crying and having it on for like five hours…so, I think I will just dive right in and tell you guys about today.

Well, it is Super Bowl Sunday, so that's a big thing. We actually went over to my grandpa's house to watch it because we don't have cable. My grandpa actually put a lot of effort into our visit even though it was just [casual], because recently, he got out of the hospital and we did find out that he has a third cancer in his pancreas…so, he wanted us to have a good gathering. So basically, he just wanted everything to be perfect. Like, my aunt bought mustard from a bottle instead of a jar, and he was like "It's wrong, you gotta take it back", and I was like, "Grandpa it's okay, I don't really like mustard!"

Um, before I got there I got all ready and I put on my clothes and all that…I was like, oh my god, I look adorable. I took so many selfies, and you can see them on my Tumblr, which I will link down below. But, um, right after I finished putting on my eyeliner I was like, I don't know, maybe I'm going to put on a second liner?

And then I fell. I fell on the bathroom floor which was extremely gross, but I'm used to it by now, and I was able to get myself up by using the toilet to, like, prop myself up…that sounds really gross…whenever I stand up, any time, out of a chair or off the couch, or whatever, I need to use my arms to lift myself up. So I was sitting there and I kept trying to stand up, and I could get about halfway, but my knees were just locked in place…I was kind of just sitting there crying and yelling at my legs, basically, like under my breath I was saying:

"You're gonna work", and I was like, "why aren't you working? Why are you doing this to me?"

The really *weird* thing about my Conversion Disorder is that I always get the weakest before I go out places. If I'm going to a doctor's appointment or a family gathering, or if I'm going to my friends house, no matter how I feel…like, I could be super pumped, like, "Oh yeah, I'm gonna go to my friend's house" or "Oh, I'm gonna see my grandpa, that's super awesome"… but somewhere my subconscious mind is just like, "No Ivy, you're staying home" and I'm just like…."No, screw you, I'm gonna go out and you're not going to stop me!"

To have to battle with my own mind is extremely frustrating and extremely tiring, and…today was just one of those days where I barely made it. I did, and I went to my grandpa's house and got a bunch of hugs and kisses. They're actually still there watching the Super Bowl and I'm at home, because we were just like…well, I feel kind of bad, because I spent about half the time trying to figure out the Wi-Fi password... I visited with my grandpa and my aunt and I saw their dogs, and their cat, and oh my god, I love them so much, I'm so jealous. Yeah, we had a really good time. I have been trying very hard to find the inspiration to write something and I finally think… I want to make more serious videos, not just, "Hi guys, I'm good. how are you?" type videos. So definitely be on the lookout for that. By Friday I want to have at least one "serious" video posted, so I'm really going to push myself to just sit down and write.

Another cool thing: if you can see in the background…look at that, wow! It's actually an art project thingy I did. I got eight CDs and I drew the phases of the Moon on them… if you want a better view of how it looks, it is on my Tumblr, which of course will be below, like always. Okay, I promised you guys an update on my legs, so, you know…the show must go on.

[switches to a shot of me sitting in a desk chair, showing my legs]
 okay so basically, I'm super weak right now, but *[kicks leg out]* look at what I can do!...I'm not feeling too great right now, but hopefully I will be feeling better by tomorrow so I can go to school. I don't know if I already told you guys this, but, I am back to doing three periods a day. It's really weird how before I was doing six periods and now I'm back to three, and that alone feels like more than [I can handle]. So, that's definitely a little discouraging, but I have promised myself that I will go to school at least once a week. Even if I miss all the rest of the days, it's alright.

I love you all so much, and you honestly just have no idea how much one comment can go towards motivating me. I absolutely love to hear other people's stories, so if you're ever going through a tough time– even if it's not about conversion disorder– if you're doing not good in school or whatever, I just really love talking to people… I'll end this video because I kind of look like a drunk raccoon, and my hair is trying really hard. I hope you guys all had a wonderful week and a great Sunday…um, tomorrow's Monday for some of you, depending on where you live, and I hope your week gets off to a good start! Mondays are always very tough, so this is your Sunday evening reminder that you can do this, and you're so strong, and you are not alone, and I believe in you, because you are amazing…I will keep you updated.

***

I uploaded a video 10 months later on **November 27th, 2015**, titled **"An update, sort of"**.

The video is 26 minutes and 40 seconds long.

It is also available to watch on my channel, along with all of the videos transcribed here. I decided to summarize this video instead of typing out a full transcription due to its length.

I apologize to my audience for going on hiatus, and give an unfortunate update…at the beginning of 2015 I made a resolution to be walking independently by the end of the year, though I have progressed to being in a wheelchair. I explain how the straw that broke the camel's back was a nasty fall I had after changing out of my nice Thanksgiving attire, leading me to break down and finally proclaim what's been on my mind: I do NOT have Conversion Disorder.

The majority of the video is me breaking down the timeline of my symptoms, starting in middle school when I began my "awkward teenager phase". At the 19 minute mark, I explain that my parents are in dismay whenever I try to tell them that I don't believe I have Conversion Disorder, because this is a condition that I can eventually "get better" from and go back to how I was before I got sick.

Though I did my best to play along and live in denial, accepting Conversion Disorder as my reality, I am finally breaking down in this video and telling the world how I feel. I explain that "By being told that I have CD, I am told that I'll be able to walk again. Someday I'll be able to drive, someday I'll have kids, someday I'll walk down the wedding aisle…being in the chair isn't what depresses me. If I'm never going to be able to walk again, I just want to be able to accept it."

I acknowledge that being in a wheelchair won't hold me back from being able to achieve incredible things in the future, but the overall uncertainty of my situation is "this huge load of false hope weighing down on me, and it's suffocating me, and I can't do it anymore".

This is the last video I made for my channel before I received a proper diagnosis refuting the Conversion Disorder claims in June of 2016.

Rose Colored Façade

Chapter 1

I can still vaguely remember leaning against a large oak tree, the bark digging into my forehead as the sun beat down on my already beet-red face. My 5th-grade teacher waited nearby with a solemn expression that would turn into a wince every few seconds as she tried to speak between by gasping sobs; "It's okay, this isn't your fault. You don't need to be so upset".

My mother pulled up in the pickup line and instinctively got out of the car once she saw the look on my teacher's face. Mom sighed and wrapped her arms around me, asking "Did it happen again? You just couldn't make it in time?" I hid my face and cried even harder out of shame and embarrassment. What kind of 5th grader comes home in wet jeans every day because they can't make it to the bathroom in time? Surely by 10 years old I should have grown out of this kind of thing!

At first, it seemed as though I was using bathroom breaks for some form of garnering attention, and my teacher would give me the same exasperated look each time I rose my hand as if to say, *again? You have asked to go to the restroom 3 times in the last hour.*

My parents stopped allowing me to go out to public places like the grocery store because the timing was always very "convenient". They would ask me "Why do you only have to pee once we're all the way on the other end of the store?" followed by, "Now I have to walk you all the way back to the front so you can go to the bathroom. I told you to go before we left!"

I was just as confused as they were, and I hated the confrontation that came along with my unexplainable bladder issues. It finally got to a point where my teachers and parents could tell that this was impeding my day-to-day life and I wasn't *gaining* anything from the attention I got every time I would piss my pants. I wasn't going to the bathroom 5 times an hour because I wanted to get out of class, I genuinely needed to pee!

So, I started to see a urologist. I remember thinking at the time that this whole experience was ungodly humiliating. What if someone from school saw me here and found out that I have to see the pee doctor? The urologist I saw then ended up following me up until I "aged out" of her pediatric practice and had to switch over to an adult urologist. She was incredibly warm and friendly and did everything she could to make me feel less ashamed of what I was dealing with. She told me about how she sees patients like me every day, with some of them being teenagers and in high school. This concept was baffling to me, like, am I really not alone in this? Who knew incontinence was such a prevalent issue?

I won't attempt to recall all the graphic details of the testing I had done by the urologist, but they presented us with two main findings: my bladder was underdeveloped in size, and it would preemptively empty itself before being full. This was causing recurring urinary tract infections. In an ultrasound of my kidneys, they found that they were functioning normally, but I had a large area of scar tissue on one of them which was a direct result of having a UTI for months on end without being treated (This scar tissue can still be seen today, though it has never caused any complications or posed as a risk to my health). During the time that we were going through all of this, my mother grew increasingly upset with what the doctors were finding.

Usually, when you have a young child developing unexplained urinary tract infections, an alarm bell will go off in the heads of health professionals, leading them to first assume the worst…there might be some sort of sexual abuse happening. Of course, the urology team did their due diligence and spoke to both me and my mom separately. *Is there anything going on at home that we need to know about? Has someone been touching you inappropriately? Is there any chance of sexual abuse going on at home or school? Was she molested in the past?*

All of these questions seemed very random to me, as I had never had another adult so much as make an inappropriate comment towards me, let alone *rape me*. They urged me to be as honest as possible, and I definitely was, but their line of questioning felt so pointed that I almost second-guessed my own truth. I think they could tell by my demeanor and whatever my mom told them that this was unlikely to be some sort of child abuse case. We started antibiotics immediately and figured this was a one-and-done sort of situation, until a few months later when I got another UTI. Then another, and another after that. I was getting constant infections because my bladder was unable to empty completely, meaning that there was old urine sitting around and piling up over time (This is caused by having a *neurogenic bladder*).

This was starting to cause a rift in my relationship with my mother because she was terrified by the implications that might be attached to these recurring UTIs. She figured that we needed to find the root of what was causing the infections, otherwise, there could be detrimental consequences. *What sort of consequences?*

Mom sat me down and explained how serious it would be if one of my doctors made a note in my file stating that they suspect my issues to be caused by some sort of abuse. She told me that they would call CPS to the house and take all 3 of us, my two brothers and I, away from her. This thought was incredibly upsetting for me to digest, and mom made sure that I knew what part I "played" in all of this.

She towered over me and strained her vocal cords as she shouted, "Do you want me to get my kids taken away? I don't want to lose my kids, Ivy!"

She went into a "problem-solving" mode, of sorts, and became obsessive over my personal hygiene. She started to sit and watch me every time I used the bathroom to make sure I wasn't wiping incorrectly, and every morning I was told to take a shower; not a "full body" kind of shower, but one where I cleaned my genitals thoroughly. I was constantly being reminded that these issues were not only my own "fault", but they were affecting everyone around me. If I didn't do the things that I needed to do to avoid catching *yet another* urinary tract infection, I could very well be tearing my entire family apart.

Even if my issues *were* self-imposed, this is quite the load to dump on a confused and scared 10-year-old.

Chapter 2

I was having a very hard time coping with my inability to hold in my pee because it still felt like such a "babyish" issue to have. My teachers at school were all made aware of my medical situation and it was decided that I could go to the bathroom as much as I needed to, no questions asked.

One time I wasn't allowed to leave during PE which resulted in me having an accident, and I'm sure the coach who refused to let me go got a major ass-chewing that day. I was terrified of confrontation and even to this day I struggle with the thought of upsetting authority figures, so I wasn't the kind of kid who would say 'screw it, I really need to use the bathroom' and get up anyways without permission. One of the other coaches had me stay behind as the rest of the classes went back inside, and this is when I was introduced to the magical world of *poise pads.*

I knew that these were different from period pads, as they were made specifically to catch urine. The coach could tell that I was embarrassed about using a product that's typically targeted towards women in their 40s and 50s, and she attempted to make me feel a bit more at ease by letting me know that she, herself, was wearing a poise pad at that very moment! Every time she sneezed or laughed, there was a chance that a little bit might come out, so she needed the pad for protection.

It made me feel better knowing that this wasn't some foreign topic that I could never talk to anyone else about. She puffed out her chest and remarked "Look at me…I'm not some old lady, right?" I laughed at this and wiped away my tears. She also told me that most adult women— especially those who have had children— will wear poise pads every once in a while. It is a very commonplace practice, I just happened to be learning about it a bit earlier than most girls.

She let me know that I was always welcome to come by her office if I needed to talk and that she always kept spare poise pads in her drawer if I needed one.

Despite having an accumulation of adults in my life that I could safely turn to during tough times, I always felt fear whenever I tried to talk to anyone confidentially. Whether it was a teacher or a doctor, no matter where I was, I felt like I could never fully open up due to the possibility of my mother finding out. I was never allowed to express frustration or despair at home, because this would illicit a sort of trauma-Olympics between mom and I.

You think *you* have it hard? How do you think all of this makes *me* feel? *Don't you ever stop to consider that I'm sad, too? You think I want to take you to all these doctors' appointments?*

Any attempts to confide in my mother resulted in pretty explosive rants and heavy guilt trips, so I adapted by bottling up my feelings for as long as I could. As I'm sure you already know, this is not exactly healthy for a developing young mind.

My mom's preferred form of communication was yelling. She was always incredibly candid about the traumatic things she went through as a child, and openly shared intimate details about the marital issues between her and my dad. These things were used by her as ammunition; by the time I was 10 years old, I was aware of the horrible physical, sexual, and psychological abuse that had been inflicted upon my mom throughout her lifetime. All of this left her in a state of being mentally unwell, and the lasting effects were always a burden that we, her children, had to shoulder.

I can't necessarily speak for how this impacted my brothers, but I will say that all three of us were conditioned into feeling extreme guilt for mom, because anything we were dealing with couldn't even come close to the horrors that our own mother had lived through. She used her trauma to continually invalidate any of our personal issues. Our thoughts and emotions were selfish because mom had surely been through worse. This led me to experience something that many survivors of verbal and psychological abuse face, and that is an overwhelming feeling of self-doubt. You think to yourself: Well, my parents never beat me, they never made me sleep in the cold garage or withheld food from me…was I really being abused? *It wasn't even that bad, right?*

My mom was not physically abusive towards us. The marks she inflicted were invisible to most and usually harbored deep within our psyche, or, the "material for my future therapist" drawer in our brains.

However, I was young, scared, and seemingly alone in all of this. I was confined to silent subservience out of fear that expressing my thoughts or feelings would be like throwing water into a hot vat of frying oil. Mom knew exactly what to say to leave permanent, life-altering burns. We were all held hostage by her rage and had to individually find ways to cope. My brothers and I all stayed put on our individual islands, while dad stood next to mom on their island and did whatever he could to disassociate long enough to make it to the end of another day.

My father was always around but never truly present, his main purpose in the household being the "breadwinner". He was like a NPC from a video game in my life, regurgitating the same few phrases and repeating basic actions. He would go to work and pay the bills, and mom did all the everyday things to keep us alive. He rarely showed us any affection that wasn't forced, and he had zero real interest in anything that didn't involve making himself feel good. Standing up for his children who were being abused by the woman he has to share a bed with at night would kick up a lot of dust…so he kept to himself, and we did our best to do the same. We were never really a "family unit", and sometimes I still wonder if such a thing even exists.

Mom would regularly remind us how horribly dad treated her in the past and how unloved he made her feel in the present. She wanted to make sure we were aware of her unhappiness, but in a way that didn't skew our view of him as a father. She made sure to always tell us "He is a bad husband, but a great father. You guys are lucky to have such a good dad!" Sometimes she would even ask him "Isn't that right, John?" to which there was only one acceptable response: a tight-lipped smile and reaffirming nod.

This thought process left me believing that I also deserved to be abused because I was just a *bad* child.

Chapter 3

At age 11 I started middle school, which is a turbulent time for almost everyone regardless of the sort of home life you have. I was still at a point where my disease had not progressed enough to become a noticeable issue, and it seemed as though I was still completely healthy aside from some issues with incontinence. Everyone has their own personal battles to face, and mine was the fact that I had to wear ginormous diaper-sized poise pads at all times in the sixth grade. It could be worse, right? *I could lose the ability to walk! Wouldn't that be a bitch?*

I only wore oversized shirts that were long enough to cover my butt or a cardigan that could conceal any lumpiness from said diaper pads. I spent every day in constant fear that someone might open my bag and see the pads, and they would immediately know that I had to wear them so I wouldn't piss my pants, because *period* pads were much more small and dainty.

The next "milestone" in the progression of my disease became apparent when I developed an abnormal gait. My mom would park in a spot that was right outside the front of the school, but there was still a short walk to reach the car whenever I was being picked up. After completing this daily routine for some time, my mom finally decided to bring something up that had been on her mind; I got in the car, and she asked:

"So…why do you walk like that?".

I had no clue what she meant by this because I never made a conscious effort to walk a certain way, so she elaborated, "You just sway your hips in a way that almost looks like, I don't know…" she hesitated, then said "you look like you're trying to do a sexy walk. I was just wondering if you even realized you were doing it." She stated this as more of an observation than anything, and I left that conversation feeling weirdly pleased. I thought to myself, *that's cool, I have a signature walk!*

Looking back at this I can tell what mom was seeing because I've watched videos of myself walking as my legs got weaker. Instead of doing heel-toe, bending-at-the-knees walking, I was using my hips to thrust my legs forward with each step. I was sauntering around like a Grand Theft Auto stripper, and everyone just assumed I was doing it on purpose.

The bottom soles of all my shoes were completely worn down because I dragged my feet horribly, due to not having the strength to lift them. I also had holes in all the knees of my jeans, because I would trip and fall constantly. I ended up becoming a regular at the nurse's office for skinned knees, and by the time I was in 8th grade she told me that she had seen my health decline over the three years I went to that school, and she always had a feeling that I needed more help than I was getting.

It always leaves a pit in my stomach when I talk to my old teachers and friends I had in middle school because they all generally say the same things: they saw me getting worse and worse over time, but no one had any idea what was actually happening. I didn't have a clear or concise way to explain why I was struggling. When they realize that I am now wheelchair bound and I was slowly deteriorating in front of their eyes for multiple years, there's a sort of pity that emits, as if they feel guilt for not doing more. As if that was even an option.

The progression of my disease was so slow and gradual that it took a while for anyone— even myself— to realize that there was something wrong. Separate from my physical health, I was struggling with a growing case of depression and anxiety. My mental health had been on a downward decline from as early as 10 years old, and I'm not sure how or when, but this eventually led me down a very dark path. I was probably 12 or slightly younger when I first started to self-harm. I can't recall a specific "reason" as to why I started hurting myself like this, but I remember that it eventually became a coping mechanism for dealing with my tumultuous home life.

I felt very misunderstood and confused (as most preteens do) about a long list of things, and I didn't have a safe outlet to talk about what was weighing on my mind.

By this time my mom and dad fought a lot less than they did when I was a kid, but there was still an unspoken agreement within the house that we all needed to tread lightly and do whatever it takes to not upset mom. It was quite frightening because mom was not always in a bad mood, her rage and outbursts were simply *pending*. The air was so thick with anticipation that it often felt hard to breathe comfortably in my own home. But mom would never STAY mad.

She would blow up, isolate herself for a bit so she could sulk privately, then emerge from her cocoon of darkness and declare everything to be "back to normal". All of this would happen in a matter of hours, maybe half a day if she was *really* upset. She would often get irritated when she would be ready to go back to rainbows-and-sunshine mode and we were still, understandably, shaken up by her tantrums. She wanted to be able to sweep everything under the rug ASAP so that she never had to address how her words or actions hurt us. There was never any sort of resolution.

I had so much pent-up sadness and anger, so I started to hurt myself as a way of relieving the extreme frustration I was feeling. I would sit on the bathroom counter at night once everyone was in bed and I knew I wouldn't be interrupted, and I would desecrate my legs. It started with simply scratching myself with my nails until I bled, then I would pound my fists against my thighs repeatedly until welts would form and I would have bruises the next day.

I always stuck to hurting my legs because they would always be covered up by pants, whereas cutting my wrists would be way too risky; I needed to stick to low-visibility areas. I didn't know how to obtain singular razor blades like all the other kids who cut themselves (thank god), so I would find other sharp objects to slice myself up with.

There was a night that I was alone in my bedroom with the door closed, and I was leaning up against a full-length mirror that was propped up against my wall at a 45-degree angle. The mirror had no frame or anything, so it was basically just a thin and fragile pane of glass that I was leaning on with all my weight. I was so focused on whatever I was doing that I didn't even have time to process it when the mirror suddenly shattered beneath me.

I looked down at the glittering fragments of glass that were dispersed throughout my bedroom carpet and started to collect the larger shards that would be easiest to throw away. As I was making a pile of all the pieces I could pick up by hand, I couldn't help but stare at the sharp edges of these reflective daggers.

The next thing I did was grab my jewelry box and hand-pick 5 or 6 of the smaller pieces of broken mirror that I would stash away for later. After that, I cleaned up the rest of the glass and went about my day. I ended up using these pieces of broken glass to scratch up my legs for a while until I was confronted by a friend's mother about my self-inflicted injuries. She must have caught a glance of my ankles/shins and realized that the pattern and placement of these cuts weren't exactly accidental.

She was driving me home from their house when she asked me about it and told me that I could always come to her if I felt like I needed help. I got flustered and told her a half-truth, saying that I had accidentally broken a mirror and now there was a bunch of glass stuck in my carpet that I kept getting scratched by. She immediately called my bullshit, in a nice way, and told me that she wanted to help.

This woman had a coop of chickens that lived in her backyard (which my mom thought was disgusting and unsanitary) so she offered to have me come along with her to the feed store so she could get supplies for her chickens and I could talk to a trusted adult for a bit…with my mother's permission, of course. I immediately went into a panic mode and told her that this would only open up a world of hurt for me; mom would immediately start speculating and become suspicious. *Why is this grown woman trying to hang out with you? Don't you see how creepy that is?*

If I tried to explain to her that I just needed some time to talk to someone about personal issues I was dealing with, then it would be, *why can't you talk to me? Why do you treat me like some kind of monster? Nobody loves me and you obviously think I'm the worst mother on the planet!*

My friend's mom could tell that I was genuinely terrified of my mother, and promised not to tell her about the cutting. Some might say this was irresponsible of her, but she could easily predict that disclosing these things to my parents would only make my home life more dangerous than it already was.

As my physical health declined over time, I started to develop a dysmorphic hatred for my legs. I hated my legs so much because they didn't work the way they were supposed to. I hated the fact that they were so weak for seemingly no reason, so my new goal was to mutilate them as a sort of "punishment". I didn't enjoy feeling pain, and I felt ill at the sight of my own blood pooling beneath me, yet, I felt as though I deserved to be suffering. I was always looking for new and inventive ways to inflict harm and pain upon myself, and at one point I ended up learning about eraser burns.

I would usually give myself eraser burns on my shins because it was a flat and hard surface that was easy to wear down, so I would aggressively scrub my legs until there were shiny, red patches of raw skin left behind. As the burns started to heal and scab over, I would immediately pick the scabs off each time, because I always heard that if you pick a scab you might end up with a scar. I desperately wanted to leave behind permanent marks on my legs so I could always look at them and remember how useless, how *worthless,* they were to me.

I can gladly report that none of this ever actually left me with permanent scarring, and I don't have any long-lasting damage to any part of my body from when I would routinely self-harm.

<u>Chapter 4</u>

Shortly after I entered the 7th grade I was given my first official diagnosis.

We were at a point where it was nearly impossible to ignore my developing weakness, though it was tough for my parents to know exactly how worried they needed to be after being blown off by my PCP countless times. This physician was ultimately the launchpad for me to be thrust into a network of healthcare providers who were all connected intrinsically and would end up deciding the fate of my medical care for the next several years.

These "doctors" were perpetually eating each other's asses, like a human centipede of like-minded individuals. My PCP stood her ground and insisted that I was simply going through a growth spurt and that my parents were looking into the matter too deeply.

I was beginning to lose my ability to balance, and I could not walk anywhere unless I had one hand on a wall or another person to hold me up. I was also so weak that I could no longer get up off the floor whenever I fell, so I required someone else to physically lift me to get back into a standing position again. This process felt especially degrading because whenever I was at school and I needed help getting off the ground, the teachers would say "Okay, let me go find one of the *strong boys* to help you". These were always guys who played on the football team, so rumors started to spread about how I would purposely act helpless in order to get the *big strong football boys* to pay attention to me.

It was the Halloween of 2013 that made mom and dad finally realize they needed to fight to get some answers. My father took my younger brother and I out that night to do some light trick-or-treating. Overall I think we walked less than a block away from our house when I collapsed onto the sidewalk and started to cry. My legs felt like cinder blocks and I simply could not walk any farther. I had pushed myself to the point of exhaustion, and it was so discouraging to know that my "breaking point" would arise after less than 10 minutes of casual walking.

None of it made any sense and I was getting very scared. I was a complete wreck and I think this was the first time my mom was able to truly recognize the fact that I was in *pain.*

I had to learn the hard way that just because we are told someone is here to help us, that it doesn't mean they will set aside their own agenda by default, even when it is the absolute right thing to do. People who we're told have good intentions still have their own self-interest intact, and this can become a very dark force which drives the decision making process of those who are meant to be the altruists of society. Think about the doctors, lawyers, people who run non-profit organizations; nobody wants to believe that a bunch of pediatric doctors would work together for years to string along a family and their sick child in order to cover up their mistakes, because...what kind of sick fuck would take part in such a thing?

<u>Why would a doctor do such severe harm, despite taking an oath to do no harm before entering the medical field?</u>

My parents chose to be willfully ignorant for as long as they could because they kept repeating the same, single question: *Why would they lie to us?*

A few days after Halloween my mom scheduled an appointment with the PCP where we planned to confront the doctor head-on, refusing to leave without some form of a solution or a plan on how to go forward with treating whatever the hell was going on with me. This time would be *different*, said mom, because we would be bringing my dad along as well. If a *man* was present it would be virtually impossible to remain overlooked!

Mom had a fear of appearing hysterical or as though she was suffering from Munchausen by proxy after persistently bringing up my worsening health, so this time she would bring "the big guns" to prove the severity of the situation.

When my mother began reciting a speech that she had been carefully rehearsing all morning, stating that something was going on with her daughter and it needed to be addressed properly, the doctor seemed utterly exasperated. She stood and listened with her hands folded and a tight-lipped expression. My dad picked up on this and reiterated everything my mom had just said but in a slightly more "assertive" tone.

Finally, before the doctor could dismiss these concerns, my mom commanded me to sit down on the floor; I sat on the ground with my legs criss-cross applesauce, looking up at the doctor with fear in my eyes. Mom stared down the pediatrician while saying "Okay, now stand back up for me. Show the doctor how hard it is for you to stand up". I struggled for a bit before ultimately needing help up off the sticky carpeted floors, and the doctor finally spoke.

She exhaled as if she was about to finally open the floodgates that she was desperately trying to keep closed all these years. "Look, I know that you have been struggling with this for a while now. At least a few years, right? It seems to only be getting worse, so I feel like we finally need to address these issues head-on and find out what is causing them". Mom let out a small sigh of relief.

"I'm going to give you some very specific instructions, and I need you to follow them exactly", my PCP told us. I tensed up as tears started rolling down moms cheeks, and we clung onto every word the doctor continued to say. This was when the very first incident of medical malpractice took place.

The pediatrician instructed my parents to take me over to the children's hospital across the street where they would be expecting us, so we could walk straight to the admissions office. She was going to call and brief them on the situation beforehand. When we got there, however, we needed to *lie* to the doctors and nurses…we would present them with a narrative that would instill a sense of urgency and make it so that I would be seen right away. This pediatrician told us that we needed to tell the hospital staff about all of my symptoms— the incontinence, abnormal gait, loss of balance, weakness in my legs— but we had to say that *all of this had started happening within the last two weeks.*

She told us that such a rapid decline in health would make the doctors at the hospital want to start doing testing immediately, whereas a situation that was as slow-progressing as mine would not ring any alarm bells, and it would likely be months before I could get in to see any sort of specialist. This made a lot of sense to my parents and even myself, at the time, so we did exactly as we were told.

<u>Chapter 5</u>

The plan unfolded perfectly and I was admitted into my own hospital bed by that evening. I was in the hospital for a whopping three days while they conducted "every test under the sun". These tests included a handful of blood tests, an MRI of my brain and entire spine with and without contrast, and a bilateral X-Ray of my knees. Unfortunately for me, all of these tests came back completely "clean". There was nothing the doctors could immediately see that would explain my symptoms. These results paired with a clinical history of *rapid onset* weakness, incontinence, and other neurological issues were enough for the medical team to conclude my first official diagnosis.

At the end of my three-day stay, we all met with *Dr. E*, the leading neurologist on my case. Another thing I had to learn the hard way is the fact that being told your doctors found *nothing* wrong with you can be just as devastating as being told that they found results of something bad, because the ambiguity of living with a "mystery illness" is truly maddening.

E entered the room along with a collection of random interns, ready for morning rounds. She was an older blonde woman with dead, icy blue eyes. Sensing our anticipation, she folded her hands and put on a wide smile.

"Well, I have great news! We weren't able to find any exact cause for the symptoms Ivy is experiencing".

My parents were already giddy with hope after hearing this, meanwhile, I felt my stomach plummet. "Based on the test results we've received and the clinical history we were given, I diagnose Ivy with Conversion Disorder".

Let me briefly explain what "Conversion Disorder" means: It causes psychological trauma to manifest physically. People with conversion disorder report symptoms such as neurogenic seizures, sudden paralysis, losing the ability to speak, and temporary blindness. There is no physiological explanation for the symptoms these people experience because the cause is rooted in mental illness.

You know the saying "It's all in your head"? Turns out they were onto something when they came up with that. We already know that our mental state has a direct effect on our physical status, like when you're nervous and your palms become clammy, or how your heart "skips a beat" when you see someone you feel romantic attraction towards. It's a simple concept, but when the effects of trauma start to cause prolonged physical impairment that limits you to the point of disability, we must classify it as a disorder. People who genuinely have Conversion Disorder do not fabricate their symptoms and experience the very real fear that comes along with losing the ability to control your body.

My mom squealed with excitement as you would expect any parent to do after being told that their child was, in fact, *not* diseased and dying. After giving us the rundown of what my treatment plan consisted of, the doctor finally broke eye contact with my parents, who were eagerly nodding along, to address me, the patient. "How does all of that sound to you?" She asked me this, not because she wanted my input and thoughts on the situation, but to make sure that I was on the same boat as the rest of them. At this point, I was crying and choking on my own words because I knew that I wasn't to express my dismay or the fact that I was dubious of the entire situation.

My mom turned her attention towards me as well and realized that I wasn't smiling along with the rest of them. She transformed instantly as if there was the flip of a switch inside her, and the joyous mother celebrating her healthy child became the disgusted parent who interpreted my negative emotions as a direct attack.

"What is wrong with you? This is the best news we could have hoped for. Why do you *want* to be sick? Why are you trying to find a problem where there isn't one?"

My mom spoke in a shrill tone and the interns seemed to tense up, avoiding looking at me for longer than a few seconds at a time, similar to how one attempts to avert their gaze from a child being berated for acting up in the middle of the grocery store.

We were discharged later that afternoon with a prescription for Prozac, a referral to physical therapy, and a 3 month follow-up appointment scheduled with Dr. E. Mom was always too self-conscious to unleash her rage in public so she would let it simmer and build up until the second she could get her victim in the safety of her own home or vehicle. My dad sat slumped over in silence as mom frantically stuffed our belongings into a duffel bag so we were ready to leave the second the green light to go was given. I knew what was coming, and I used this time to mentally prepare.

She was so upset that the anger started to boil over during the elevator ride down to the main floor, mumbling "How dare you", over and over while shaking her head disapprovingly. She made sure we were out of the parking lot before finally letting the show begin. Dad kept his mouth shut and eyes forward while mom wailed between accusatory insults and I sobbed for the entirety of the short ride home.

Chapter 6

By this time I was not only trying to prove that I was sick, but that I was not *pretending* to be sick. Growing up I was never known to fake being sick to get out of going to school like most kids do at one point or another, because I actually preferred being there far more than staying at home. The first person to plant the liar-liar-pants-on-fire seed in my mother's mind was my physical therapist, T.

I remember stepping onto the treadmill for the first time and thinking, *hey, I could get used to this!* I was able to hold onto the railings on each side which eliminated the need to focus on my balance and I could choose the speed I was walking at. Mom felt so inspired by this that she went ahead and bought a treadmill for the house, saying "We can all get some use out of this!" Mom used the treadmill less than a dozen times. I was the only one who used it, typically while listening to my iPod on full blast so I could block out the burning pain in my legs. I hated that fucking treadmill.

I also did an exercise where I would stand on a curved balance board while throwing a basketball against a trampoline about 5 feet in front of me, then catching the ball when it propelled back my way. This one was pretty stressful and I would only do it if someone stood nearby to serve as a handheld if I fell over (which resulted in numerous accidental groping incidents). With PT twice a week and my weekly sessions with a mental health counselor, my parents were told to expect integral improvement in my ability to walk, so long as I was fully committed to the treatment plan. I was constantly reminded by mom and healthcare workers that the only person who could fix this mental illness and the effect it was having on my body was *me*, so I better be ready to put in the work.

Even though I still had a sneaking suspicion that this was not conversion disorder, the only way I could survive was to effectively brainwash myself into accepting the mind-over-matter rhetoric that was being shoved down my throat. I desperately wanted to be normal again. I spoke about this quite a bit on my Instagram.

These things are much easier said than done, of course, but I was still working my ass off with very minimal results. After months of watching me get weaker, the physical therapist pulled my mom aside and let her know that she believed I was not taking the program seriously enough, and that I was actually faking my decline in health. Someone who was genuinely working on getting better both mentally *and* physically would not be getting weaker over time.

Supposedly there were more than enough "inconsistencies" marked in my chart by that point to back up this theory, and the physical therapy team collectively decided that they would not be renewing my referral once I ran out of insurance-approved appointments with them. They told my mom that I was taking up a spot that could be filled by a child who was actually in need.

01/14/2014 - TREATMENT in Physical Therapy Department (continued)

Notes (continued)

			O-Ongoing M=Met D=Discontinued	
In 2 months, Ivy will be able to walk without deficits and normal cadence to allow her to be able to go from class to class in allotted amount of time.	Scissoring and crouched pattern, slow cadence	11/26/2013	Ongoing	1/3/14 better heel strike when focusing on gait, continues with decreased knee extension stability 1/7/14 unchanged 1/10/14 pre session, slight knee flexion but getting heel strike consistently; post session, more knee flexion and lower dorsiflexion but still achieving heel strike most of the time 1/14/14 more knee flexion today overall
In 2 months, Ivy will increase B LE strength to 5/5 without any "giving" during testing.	Hip flex 3+; Hip AD/AB 4/5; Knee ext 3/5; knee flex 4/5; DF 4+; PF 3/5	11/26/2013	Ongoing	1/3/14 knee ext static 5/5 but effort to get to full extension 1/7/14 supportive therex 1/10/14 supportive therex 1/14/14 supportive therex
In 2 months, Ivy will be able to perform single leg stance >10 sec R and L to improve balance.	~3 sec R and L	11/26/2013	Ongoing	1/3/14 supportive therex 1/7/14 supportive therex 1/10/14 supportive therex 1/14/14 supportive therex

PAIN
Numeric Rating Scale: 0/10

EDUCATION
Treatment session was observed by mother. Explanation was provided. Understanding was verbalized by mother and patient.

ASSESSMENT
Complained about exercises throughout session today, reports being tired. Performed all exercises as given but did appear to fatigue more quickly today.

PLAN
Continue treatment - 2 times per week. Discussed decreasing to 1X week soon.

Start Time of Therapy: 8:10
End Time of Therapy: 8:50
Length of Session: 40 minutes

02/25/2014 - TREATMENT in Physical Therapy Department (continued)

Notes (continued)

Treatment Goal	Baseline	Start Date	Status O-Ongoing M=Met D=Discontinued	Daily Progress
In 2 months, Ivy will be able to walk without deficits and normal cadence to allow her to be able to go from class to class in allotted amount of time.	Scissoring and crouched pattern, slow cadence	11/26/2013	Discontinue goal	2/4/14 improved knee extension, heel strike and cadence but still reverts to flexed gait at times 2/11/14 more flexed today 2/18/14 less flexed LE's and better heel strike noted today 2/25/14 more knee flexion noted today; when reminded, able to get near full knee extension Discontinue goal
In 2 months, Ivy will increase B LE strength to 5/5 without any "giving" during testing.	Hip flex 3+; Hip AD/AB 4/5; Knee ext 3/5, knee flex 4/5; DF 4+, PF 3/5	11/26/2013	Discontinue goal	2/4/14 supportive therex; abd 3/5, add 3/5 2/11/14 supportive therex; overall 2-3/5 2/18/14 supportive therex 2/25/14 unchanged from 2/4 Discontinue goal
In 2 months, Ivy will be able to perform single leg stance >10 sec R and L to improve balance.	~3 sec R and L	11/26/2013	Discontinue goal	2/4/14 supportive therex 2/11/14 unable to perform more than 1-2 seconds 2/18/14 unchanged 2/25/14 1-2 seconds Discontinue goal

PAIN
Numeric Rating Scale: 0/10

EDUCATION
Caregiver remained in lobby during the session. Explanation was provided. Understanding was verbalized by mother. Mom reports as soon as their insurance is renewed she will seek counseling for Ivy. Also still considering return to Dr.

ASSESSMENT
Worked well. Gait regressed intermittently today with more knee flexion and buckling. Performs all exercises well. Ivy has made minimal progress over the course of this therapy episode but up and down and recently some slight regression of gait noted. Patient initially not performing HEP or recommendations at home but recently has been more compliant and is also using a treadmill that the family purchased. Patient in need of some counseling in light of diagnosis but parent somewhat resistant initially due to fear of patient being medicated. Recent discussions with mom

105

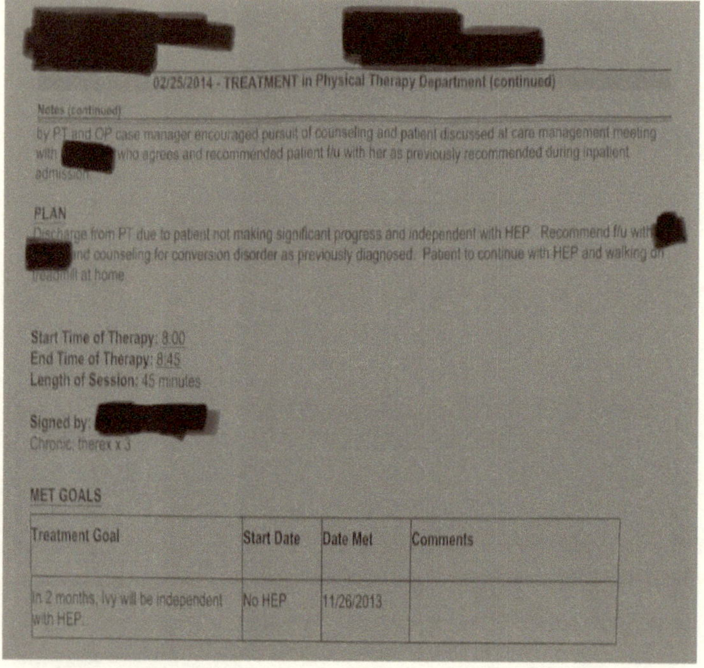

Treatment Goal	Start Date	Date Met	Comments
In 2 months, Ivy will be independent with HEP.	No HEP	11/26/2013	

Notice the dates of these two appointments; within a month and a half, the physical therapy team was ready to drop me due to "lack of progress".

My first therapist never outright said that she felt like I was "faking" everything, but she shared similar sentiments. After I got past the fear that my mom would be able to hear what I was saying through the walls, I felt very comfortable talking with D. She was very soft-spoken and did her best to gently ease into heavier topics that weren't easy to talk about. I went into therapy knowing that I was there to answer one looming question: What caused me to develop Conversion Disorder?

Sometimes I would lay in bed at night and think about what would happen, hypothetically, if I came up with a lie to get everyone off my back. *Maybe my dad would take me out into the garage and beat me every night, or perhaps my older brother had been molesting me for years and forced me to live in silence.* The thought of claiming such terrible things, even if it was to make my life easier, made me feel nauseous. I knew I could never go through with it, but I considered it more than once.

Mom liked to do her own prodding to help speed things along, so to speak, after I had been going to therapy regularly for months without even a glimpse of a breakthrough. Every few weeks or so she would sit me down on the couch in a very ceremonious fashion and say things like "You know you can tell me anything, right? You can trust me. If something happened to you that I don't know about, I won't get angry when you tell me. I promise."

These interrogation sessions never ended well; it would always lead to me crying, and her screaming at me for withholding such important information from her, *my own mother*.

I would break down out of frustration every time because I simply didn't have the answer she was looking for. There was no repressed trauma buried deep in my psyche that was so horrendous it was literally crippling me. Before my diagnosis, I was a very regular child living a very decent life. I had a mentally ill mom and an emotionally detached father, sure…but I was so normal that it was a privilege.

One time on the way to therapy, my mom wanted to help me brainstorm things I should talk about. I saw her eyes light up before blurting out "I know! Remember that one time I was so angry at your dad that I ripped your Rapunzel poster off the wall? You were heartbroken, you really loved that poster." I started laughing out of pity and told her that I didn't even remember this happening until she brought it up. It was a traumatic incident, for sure, but I never lost sleep over it or anything.

I brought this up in therapy, anyways, and D was so delighted she almost fell out of her chair as she went to grab her EMDR machine. She had me close my eyes and put one pulsator in each hand, focusing on the feeling of them buzzing back and forth.

D: "Now, put yourself back in that moment…what emotions were you experiencing? How did you *feel?*"

Me: "I felt…sad? Like I wanted to cry?"

D: "How do you feel about this event now? Are you still feeling those same emotions?"

Me: "I guess not. I don't really care about the poster. But what a bitch, right? Maybe she's the one who should be here, not me! Haha!"

Needless to say, we never got very far with EMDR.

<u>Chapter 7</u>

"Smile big, show me your teeth. Stick out your tongue. When I touch your face, does it feel the same on both sides?"

I f I had a dollar for every routine neuro check I've sat through…well, you get the joke.

My parents were loyal, unwavering fans of Dr. E. They took everything she said at face value, because what else were they supposed to do? Communicate with their sick child? *We don't do due diligence in this house.* Every three months we would report to the same pediatric neurology clinic to follow up with the same pediatric neurologist who gave me, a pediatric patient with no recorded history of mental illness, the official diagnosis of "Conversion Disorder".

I held my breath and sat like a good little statue with Dr. E so close to my face that I was afraid she might poke one of my eyes out. As she shined a flashlight in my eyes I looked straight ahead, up, left, right, and down so many times in a row that my eyeballs felt fatigued. She took a step back and looked at me with a deep frown. "Let me…try something", she mumbled, before switching off the overhead lights.

She repeated the same directions as before and I happily obliged; she had to have seen something. Why would she be taking this long if she didn't? She backed away again, slower this time, and turned the lights back on unceremoniously. I could sense my mom's hesitation to speak, simply uttering "So…what is it?"

The doctor clasped her hands in front of her and grinned. "All good! I'll see you again in three months". Hooray. You know that sound a balloon makes after you poke a small hole in it and it deflates slowly? Stuttered, almost stifled shrieks as the air rushes to escape from the minuscule exit…I felt like that balloon.

The neurologist was well aware of the continuous, developing weakness in my legs. It never sat right with me how self-assured they were in my diagnosis, and how vehemently they denied to do any sort of further tests. My PCP had regular correspondence with Dr. E and let her know each time we would bring this up at regular doctors' appointments, so Dr. E could give my mother and I the same scolding speech at our next neurology appointment:

Ivy has Conversion Disorder. Ivy is mentally unwell and she can not get better if we enable her. There is no logical reason that Ivy can not walk right now. Do not listen to Ivy, listen to her doctors.

According to all of my doctors, I was most definitely faking this. This made my parents look bad because it meant that they must have been coddling me and raising a sick little liar who would do anything for attention. Regardless, my legs were getting weaker and I struggled to get around the house without falling. Mom went online and bought me a shiny new quad-foot cane; I even got to pick the color, which was blue. She studied me as I attempted to walk in a straight line with the cane, but I was feeling very off-balanced.

Mom grabbed the cane to show me how I was using it, versus how I was supposed to be using it. I needed to learn how to coordinate using the cane with each step and lean on it for support. I looked a lot like an actor who landed the role of a character who walks with a cane, yet never figured out how to believably use the mobility aid. I was disappointed because I thought the cane would grant me so much more independence, but I still felt like I was constantly on the verge of falling.

This was right around the time mom made another exciting purchase: a brand new dishwasher. We always had an old dishwasher that was installed, but it didn't work for some reason, so we could never actually use it. Mom decided to finally bite the bullet and replace the appliance, and we were all looking forward to it. No more scrubbing or hand-washing for us! Mom was the one who did the dishes the most, though, and we were happy to see her buying something that would make her life easier.

Mom is the type of person to excessively deny herself any comfort or luxury, no matter how small, so that she can constantly remind the people around her how much she sacrifices for them (out of the goodness of her own heart, of course). She must be the biggest victim who has suffered the most in any and all situations, and you are inherently indebted to her because of that fact.

I was sitting on the living room couch when she called my name with one foot out the back door, "Ivy, I need you to empty the dishwasher for me". I hoisted myself up and grabbed my handy-dandy cane so I could wobble over to the kitchen. I clutched onto the edge of the counter as I bent over at the waist to pick up the dishes, knees locked and straight so they wouldn't give out underneath me.

I either lost my grip or pushed my luck while reaching across to grab some silverware because I ended up toppling over the open door of the dishwasher. Mom came rushing inside when she heard the loud crash and found me laying half on the floor, half on the door of the dishwasher.

I kept saying "It's okay, I'm okay, I'm fine" in an attempt to deescalate the situation, but that wasn't what mom was focused on…she was frozen in place, muttering "You just broke my new dishwasher. It's fucked now". At first, I thought she was being dramatic, but once I was able to get up off the ground we attempted to close the dishwasher. It wouldn't latch shut. Unfortunately, the hinges were not designed to hold this amount of weight; the new dishwasher *was* broken.

I was mortified by how expensive of an accident this was and crushed when I saw the look on my mom's face. She finally got *one* thing, and I had ripped it out from underneath her.

When I started to cry it enraged her. She threw her hands up and said "You know what? Now I know. I won't ask you to help with anything around the house anymore". I stared at her blankly for a moment before she said "You will do anything to get what *you* want, and I am done letting you ruin everything because of it". My mother thought so little of me as a person, of my character, that she believed I broke her brand new dishwasher because I wanted to get out of doing my chores.

My sole purpose, in my mothers' eyes, was to live life in spite of her.

Chapter 8

I would spend quite a lot of time sitting in the bathroom alone with my thoughts because I felt like I could get the most privacy there. Back when I was still strong enough to do so, I would boost myself up onto the counter and sit cross legged in front of the mirror for extended periods of time, usually until my legs went numb. I always just hoped that my family would assume I was taking a massive dump and leave me to ruminate.

The specific details leading up to what I'm going to talk about next are fuzzy at best, and I'm assuming that's because my brain has done its best to block the event out completely. I was one of those kids who would brag about never breaking a bone before, like I was part of some exclusive club…a club that I lost membership to on this day.

As I slowly lowered myself off the countertop, I made the grave mistake of keeping one hand on my cane for support. The metal rod wobbled as I leaned onto it with my full body weight and I managed to take two panicked steps forward before tripping over the dingy lilac bath mat. This wasn't my first fall in the bathroom; I would routinely fall when getting up off the toilet, and I spent hours finding different ways to get back up on my own after mom banned my brothers and father from helping me. She told them that they needed to stop enabling me when I fell and the only way I would get better was if I was forced to help myself.

The tile was ice cold but I still broke out into a full-body sweat. When I fell, my left foot stayed trapped underneath me. There was a distinct *crack* followed by dull, searing pain. *I fucked up. I fucked up. Mom is going to be so pissed.* I just laid there for a few minutes while weighing my options, but I simply didn't have the courage to look at the damage. I took one last shaky breath before calling out, "Mom…I need you to come here". I listened as she got up out of her recliner, left her bedroom, and made her way down the hall towards me.

"Did you fall again?" she asked casually. I heard her begin to turn the doorknob and I panicked even more.

"Stop, stop! Don't…" I was going to say "Don't come in," because I wanted to prepare her for what she was about to see.

I lowered my voice and said, "well, I think I broke something. I think something is wrong". Mom took a pregnant pause.

"Okay, sweetie…I'm going to open the door". When she saw one leg straight and the other pretzeled under my body, she spoke slowly as she said "You have to let me look. We need to straighten your leg". I nodded and let out choked sobs until she realized what she was looking at.

"John, I need you to get in here RIGHT NOW!" She summoned both my older brother and father. I glanced at the carpet next to me and saw red spots, then I slowly scanned over my left leg…at the very end, to my complete horror, I realized I was missing the tip of my pinky toe. It dangled by a thin piece of skin perpendicular to a shard of bone sticking up and out. At this point I wasn't crying because I was in pain, but because I was terrified of whatever was going to happen next.

My father grabbed me under my arms and my brother scooped up my lower half so they could jointly carry me out to the car. My poor brother was hyperventilating the entire time, and I caught a peek of dad's "I'm going to vomit" face as he laid me down in the back seat of our Dodge minivan.

I spent the ride to the ER gasping for air and apologizing an inappropriate number of times while mom and dad assured me it was going to be fine, and we would fix this. I remember being too afraid to lay eyes on the injury, but when we got there, the admitting nurse took one look at it and said "Ouch! Looks like you had an accident, huh?" I really miss being treated by pediatrics sometimes.

After a doctor reset the bone, we sat and processed what the hell just happened and waited to hear what was next. "Well…I think all the pain you just went through should be punishment enough. That must have hurt like a *bitch*!" mom joked, and I laughed half-heartedly. When she wasn't being cruel or petty, she had a lighthearted demeanor that always left me coming back for more, no matter how much she hurt me. For such a brief period of time, I think my mom felt empathy for what I was going through. For once, I wasn't the only one who felt afraid.

After some X-Rays, it was determined that I had a compound fracture, and it was bad enough to warrant surgery. The doctors even decided to put me in a cast that went all the way up to the knee, which still sounds excessive to me, but I decided to just enjoy the experience of having a cast that all my friends and family could sign…except, we were on summer break, and my family wasn't necessarily excited to be around me. Nevertheless, when I was presented with color swatches for the cast, I picked green.

***

XR TOE 1 VIEW LEFT
Collected on July 21, 2014 9:02 AM
Exam: Single view toe.
History: Trauma.
Findings: A single view of the fifth toe on the left foot demonstrates that a reduction as attempted. There remains subluxation of the proximal interphalangeal joint. Soft tissue swelling is seen.
Impression: 1. Subluxation of the proximal interphalangeal joint.

***

When I woke up from surgery there was a nurse who showed us the walking-boot attachment that I was given so that I could continue to ambulate normally. My mom interjected angrily and asked "You really expect her to walk around with that? What if she falls again and breaks another bone? She needs a wheelchair!" This prompted a visit from the surgeon who fixed my toe.

He listened to my mom with an annoyed look on his face and finally replied "You know what? If she breaks another bone, I will fix it. She is not leaving this hospital in a wheelchair, and that is a promise". He made sure to look at me as he told my parents this, and by that point, we were all beside ourselves.

Before mom's hysteria could escalate any further, the surgeon asked her and my father to come with him to his office for a private chat. I sat in the hospital room alone for a few minutes before one of the nurses came in so I could confide in her. These are two separate reports written by this nurse after I was discharged from the hospital:

***

Entered room at appx. 0725 this AM accompanied by Dr. [Redacted] and charge nurse,[Redacted]. [Redacted], PCT, also present.

Patient's mother expressed concern about some marks that the patient reportedly had to her cheeks after surgery last night. The mother stated that they resembled finger marks and was concerned that "something happened during surgery". Dr. [Redacted] reassured the patient's mother that nothing out of the ordinary occurred in OR and mentioned that her face appears fine this AM (no marks noticeable aside from a small abrasion below the patient's right eye). Patient's mother began crying and was visibly upset.

She voiced multiple concerns, including the marks to her daughter's face, a possible allergic reaction that may have occurred last PM, and her daughter's ability to move/ walk post-operatively. Discussed ambulating with the assistance of a walker, but the patient's mother stated "what if she falls and breaks a hip?" and asked if the patient could have a wheelchair. Dr. [Redacted] explained that this is a necessary risk in order to preserve the patient's mobility and aid in her recovery. The patient's mother continued to grow more agitated throughout this exchange. The patient was also visibly upset throughout this; she was noted to be crying in bed.

When asked what was the matter, the patient refused to answer. However, during my time spent in the room on this first interaction (appx. 35 minutes), the patient mouthed to me multiple times that she wanted to speak with me alone. After Dr. [Redacted] and[Redacted], RN, left the room, the patient's mother continued sobbing and even sinking to the ground to sob on the floor multiple times.

Attempted reassuring the patient's mother and addressing her concerns; however, she primarily spoke of how all of this was "very stressful on [her'" and that she "couldn't take it anymore". The patient's tearfulness and anxiety increased as her mother continued crying and discussing multiple aspects of the patient's ongoing illness. At one point, the patient stated, "Mom, you said that I ruined your life", to which her mother explained that their family's lives have become complicated and stressful "with multiple doctors visits and appointments"; she did not refute saying this to the patient.

I attempted multiple times to encourage the patient's mother to leave the room to "cool off' or "get some air", both for her own sake and for the patient's sake, but she refused stating "I won't leave her side". [Redacted] with patient relations and [Redacted] with social work were both paged at this time and [Redacted], RN, was updated on all of these events.
Electronically signed by [Redacted], RN at 7/22/2014 11:12 AM
***

(continued)

Throughout this morning, the patient continued to mouth & whisper to me that she wanted to speak with me alone. Tried multiple times to have the patient's parents leave the room, but they wanted to stay by the patient. During a meeting with [social workers], I was able to speak with the patient privately for appx. 10-15 minutes. She began to cry and stated that she "couldn't take it anymore". I asked what she was referring to and she stated, "I know my mom loves me and cares about me and I'm grateful for everything she does for me, but she blows up at me a lot and tells me really mean things".

I asked what type of things the patient was referring to and she stated, "She tells me I'm a burden and that I've ruined my family's lives and she even told me this morning that I am God's punishment for her". I questioned the patient how often her mother speaks to her like this and she said that it happens "a lot, especially when she [the patient's mother] gets angry". She also stated that her mother always apologizes afterward. I asked whether she feels safe at home multiple times and she responded that she does feel safe, but that she feels overwhelmed with many of the "mean things" her mother tells her. She also mentioned that she tried discussing these issues with her mother in the past, but her mother became very angry, threw her tea at the patient, and told her she was going to have to go live with her aunt.

Again, her mother later apologized. Asked the patient whether she wants to hurt herself and she stated "I hit myself in the thighs sometimes because I can't yell or get upset or my mom will get mad". I asked if this leaves marks, and she stated that it leaves bruises at times. I asked whether she thinks of killing herself and she stated, " sometimes think about it but would never do it" She stated she would never kill herself because it would hurt her girlfriend, [Redacted], feelings and because she doesn't want to lose her iPod. I asked whether she has people she feels like she can talk to and she stated that she is able to discuss all of these issues with her counselor, [Redacted], and her girlfriend, [Redacted]. I asked the patient if there was anything I could do for her now and she said no. All of this was relayed to [Redacted] with social work

Electronically signed by [Redacted], RN at 7/22/2014 12:17 PM
***

When my parents finally came back they had solemn looks on their faces as the surgeon told me "We have decided that you can have a walker". My mom stared past me with a disgusted scowl. After the surgeon left us alone once again, mom pulled up a chair to sit at my bedside.

There was a sour look on her face as she started to speak, saying "You know, you have a reputation around here. The surgeon spoke with Dr. E, and he knows all of your history". My stomach sank at the thought of Dr. E being the one to write my narrative.

"He really opened my eyes, Ivy. When Dr. E told me you were faking this, I wasn't so sure…but now, I can tell that you are clearly manipulating me. I won't let you." This wasn't exactly a conversation where I was allowed to pitch in, so I just sat and listened to mom tell me her new-found truth.

"He told me all about kids like you who hurt other people to get what they want. I told him about the incident with the dishwasher, and he laughed! It's direct proof that you are doing all of *this* because you are defiant. You know how much I love you, and you use that weakness to get away with things".

There are no words to describe the immense pain I felt in my chest as I listened to my mother tell me what a manipulative, ungrateful monster she thought I was. The entitled brat that *everyone* had decided I was. I was stripped of any and all integrity.

My dad didn't say a single thing; he let mom run the show, as per usual. Mom became more frantic as she continued relaying the surgeon's message, telling me "He told us that you can't have a wheelchair, because that would mean giving in to what *you* want. I refuse to enable you by letting you completely give up so you can spend the rest of your life as a 'disabled' person. I just won't have it!"

So that was that. I was sent home with a medical-grade walker and a screw in my left pinky toe that I had to hobble around with for the next 6 weeks.

Chapter 9

I'll always remember the first time I was admitted to a psychiatric hospital, though I had a total of 4 hospitalizations for suicidal ideation and attempts. The other 3 stays are a blur to me. I was still getting used to life with a walker and trying my best to stay optimistic about my next big milestone: I would be starting high school in only a few weeks!

My mom brushed me off the first few times I tried to talk to her about it until the time came for me to pick out my schedule. I read out my options, placing giddy check marks next to anything that piqued my interest.

"What do you think? I'm obviously going to take all AP courses, right? I'm not sure what kind of extracurricular classes I want to take. A few of my friends are interested in debate and I think that could be a lot of fun."

Mom let out a bitter scoff. "You aren't being serious, are you?" I hesitated before asking her what was wrong, which triggered her to snatch the pre-registration form out from under my pen. I became ridged and tried to brace myself for whatever was coming, but it was worse than I could have predicted.

"You are not going to school like that. How are you supposed to get to your classes without someone to help you if you fall? What if you're too weak?" I hadn't thought of these things until that moment, but she was right. I started to get choked up as I tried to defend my failing body, "I think I can do it. I want to go to school. I have to go to school, actually", I said meekly.

She grabbed my walker and flung it across the dining room so she could stand directly in front of me, glaring daggers through my forehead.

"Here's what's going to happen. You want to go to [redacted high school] so badly? Then we will get you put in Special Ed. You'll sit in one room all day and get all of your work brought to you. You want to *act* like a retard, you will be *treated* like a retard. It's either that or homeschool, and I don't want to homeschool you!"

Well, I wouldn't want you to homeschool me, anyways. "You'll be like those adults who don't even start high school until their twenties because they're mentally fucked in the head. *That* is what will be happening."

The thought of having my education compromised was genuinely heartbreaking. I was always academically competitive and I couldn't imagine a future that didn't involve going to college and all that jazz I had convinced myself I needed to do in order to become a respectable and successful member of society. Being held back in any capacity wasn't an option; I would sooner take my own life than endure the embarrassment of being behind all my peers developmentally (which is ironic, considering the fact that my teenage years were ravaged by an underlying illness that slowly disabled me).

I sobbed and begged my mom to let me try regular classes and she screamed at me until I gave up. I felt so helpless, and my future was beginning to look incredibly bleak. With my world quickly crumbling around me, I started mentally deteriorating at a scary rate.

The only thing scarier to me than a future as a 25-year-old highschooler was the thought of no future at all. I spent more nights than not thinking about various ways to end it all, and sometimes I wouldn't get any sleep because I spent hours trying to hype myself up enough to *just do it already*. I went back and forth on the kind of note I would leave; should I keep it short and sweet, or should I write a 10-page manifesto listing my every last grievance before I go? Which one would pack a better punch?

"I'm thinking about killing myself. I don't know if I can do this anymore." The first step is to say it out loud, I figured.

I was already expecting the flood of anger that was unleashed, but I didn't really know what was supposed to happen next. This was my cry for help. I faced both of my disheveled parents and pleaded for help because I didn't exactly *want* to die, but I definitely didn't want to be alive anymore, either.

"Well, that's just fucking great. Pack the car, John. We have to take her to [redacted behavioral hospital]."

Mom threw socks and random pairs of pants to me while I cried silently and stuffed my belongings in a duffel bag. She spent the car ride there saying things like "I hope this makes you happy. You really do always get what you want, no matter who it hurts". I felt more like a criminal in the back of a police car than a teenage girl who was getting the help she desperately needed.

As we pulled into the parking lot my mom cackled bitterly and said "I forgot they have a pool here, I should have packed your bathing suit! I bet you're going to have a fuckin' blast swimming with all your new friends". Mental illness runs quite rampant in my moms' side of the family, so this wasn't her first rodeo when it came to dropping people off at the psych ward. I spent what was supposed to be my first day of high school in a behavioral hospital.

The intake process was tedious and felt more humiliating than anything. When they asked me why I was there, I told them I wanted to kill myself. They asked me if I had a plan, and when I said yes, both of my parents raised their eyebrows at me.

"What do you mean, have you put thought into this?" Mom asked in an incredulous tone.

"Well, I took one of Dad's belts. It's in my closet. I thought I might hang myself." Dad looked more grim than ever. Saying my plan out loud made everything feel terrifyingly real.

Later on while we were back in the waiting room, mom randomly asked, "Wait, isn't that how Robin

Williams killed himself? You got the idea from him, didn't you?" She said this sarcastically and with a smirk, like it was a funny joke and I hadn't realized it yet (she was right, though. I did get the idea from him). Her attitude surrounding the situation seemed to soften as if this wasn't her child wanting to commit suicide, but just a dumb and young kid who was poorly influenced by a celebrity death.

I know that some of you are waiting to hear all the "crazy psych ward" stories I have, but it truly isn't *like the movies*. There is one main lesson I learned after all my stays in the behavioral hospital: you don't go there to feel like you no longer want to hurt yourself or others, you go there so that you simply *don't*. I'm sure plenty of people have left these inpatient grippy-sock-vacations feeling a million times better than they did before, but the real healing and treatment tends to be more of an outpatient kind of thing.

At my facility, we would each get to see one of the on-site psychiatrists every weekday for about 5 to 10 minutes. They are not there to counsel you or learn your whole life story; their job is to medicate appropriately and get the ball rolling when it comes to referring patients to any sort of outpatient-related services.

My psychiatrist was always the same guy, Dr. F, a favorite amongst the nurses. He was only a little kooky (for lack of better words) and seemed to have a genuine desire to help people. His slicked-back gray ponytail, sun-damaged skin, and gravelly voice made his white doctor's coat look out of place, as if he grabbed it off a random hook and snuck into the office "Catch Me If You Can"(2002) style.

"Why is it that you are so unhappy, miss Ivy?" the old hippie stared at me over his thick prescription glasses.

I'm sure I rambled on about a few things in an attempt to answer this loaded question, but the general consensus was that my mother would not listen to me or my feelings. I felt trapped by my own body which was failing due to the Conversion Disorder, and my inability to get better had caused my parents to resent me.

"I have treated many people with Conversion Disorder before, and let me tell you…they all got better! This is not a permanent problem. We just need to dig deep enough to find what treatment will best suit you."

Oh, great. I always wanted to be a princess or a ballerina when I grew up, not a fucking archaeologist. I was tired of listlessly digging.

"Miss Ivy…have you ever tried hypnosis?", the doctor whispered, his eyes sparkling.

Sure, I had tried listening to YouTube videos of positive subliminal affirmations in the past, but I never saw the rapid muscle growth or super-human strength that they all promised to produce. I would lay in bed with my earbuds in (because listening to these things out loud would be embarrassing) and I would mistake the tingling in my hands and legs as some sort of hypnotic spell taking over my body; it turns out my limbs were just falling asleep on me.

Dr. F had a twinkle in his eye, and the accompanying nurses all clutched their badges with anticipation, as though they were about to watch a David Blaine performance.

"Ivy, you will watch my pendulum as it swings back and forth, and you must focus on my voice completely." Yes, he went all in with the swinging pocket watch and everything.

After a minute or two of some generic mantra about overcoming my anxiety, I was instructed to close my eyes so that I could really *visualize* the next part. Dr. F inhaled deeply as one nurse put a hand on my shoulder, when he said:

"Miss Ivy…I need you to imagine yourself standing up to your mother. You are standing in front of her without the walker, and you yell: I can! I can go to school! You are stomping your feet and telling her that you WILL get better from this Conversion Disorder! Do it now!"

I hesitated for a moment, asking "Are you sure I should be yelling in here? The people outside might hear it and…you know, worry about…" I trailed off, but he was insistent.

"Yes, the door is closed, nobody is going to interrupt. Yell at your mom and stomp your feet to show her how strong you *really* are."

I shouted half-heartedly and mustered all my strength to do a couple of pathetic foot taps. "Why are you not stomping, are you scared?" I opened my eyes and glared at the psychiatrist, wishing I could say *"No, you dumbass. I can't stomp my feet. I can barely even walk, you fucking moron".*

I believe he was hoping to have one of those televangelist-style moments where the sad paralyzed subject is magically healed through the power of Jesus Christ, except my savior would be him and his impeccable hypnosis skills. When I didn't kick my walker to the side and proudly strut out of his office, he was visibly disappointed. "I want you to continue journaling. Use this time to document all of your thoughts and negative emotions so that you can work through them while you are here", he instructed.

After this "session", the nurses gushed about how brilliant Dr. F is and reminded me how lucky I was to be under his care. I didn't keep any of my journals from my time inpatient, which was probably due to the fear that mom might find them and read them. I did, however, discover my love for creating collages and vision boards from magazine clippings! Sometimes I'll cut out pictures for craft purposes and giggle at the ridiculous memory I have of making collages while in the psych ward; there was one nurse with one pair of scissors who would circle the group and cut out our chosen pictures for us.

It's not really a laughing matter (wanting to kill yourself), but isn't it just a little bit funny in hindsight? I am inexplicably glad I never went through with it. I am so incredibly happy to be alive today.

Chapter 10

For as long as I can remember, I absolutely adored my mom. One time when I was in second or third grade, a couple of reporters for the local newspaper came in to ask a few of the kids what they were thankful for that upcoming Thanksgiving. I gave them my best show-stopping smile and went home that day thinking, *I'm going to be famous!* A week or so later, our neighbor stopped by to tell us that she saw me in the paper and wanted to give us a clipping from her copy for us to keep; maybe we could frame it, or put it up on the fridge.

I scanned the rows of my fellow classmates who reported being thankful for things like their pets, their video games, the snacks their parents buy for them…I was kicking myself wishing I had thought of those things! When prompted, I told the friendly journalists the very first thing that came to mind as they knelt down to ask me: "What are you thankful for this year?"

We found this scrap of newspaper many, many years later when mom was cleaning out her bedside nightstand. Underneath piles of handmade birthday and

Mother's Day cards from years before, I found a picture of my younger self, beaming brightly, with a caption that read: *I'm thankful for my mommy.*

After leaving the behavioral hospital for the first time, we decided to try a new therapist. Luckily for me, Dr. F was able to refer me to an outpatient therapist that actually worked for the hospital; even better, she spent the first few decades of her career as a mental health nurse who worked under Dr. F himself. Sounds promising! Her name was Molly. Molly was around Dr. F's age and was clearly a seasoned veteran when it came to dealing with the craziest of the crazies.

I worried that I may come across as too "complex" of a case, but she made sure I knew my place right from the start. Mom got to sit in for our first session while we got to know each other on the surface, and I was generally hopeful that someone as experienced as her could help me in a way that would be truly meaningful. Molly was blunt and expressed her determination to work me out of having Conversion Disorder, as she had done with patients in the past.

When we left that day, mom had a pep in her step that I hadn't seen in a long time. She jabbered excitedly the whole way home, saying "I like her, like, REALLY like her! She has the tough-love sort of approach that I think you need".

Maybe I *did* need someone to give me a swift (but caring) kick in the ass to start healing, I thought. It turns out that my mother loved Molly as much as she did because they both shared the same idea of what "tough love" should look like: bullying in the name of building character.

Molly had one of those jumbo Yankee candles that smelled like maple pancake syrup and a dimly lit office with a window that gave us a perfect view of the entrance to the behavioral hospital. So very comforting, and not at all unnerving; it was like an unspoken reminder that warned people to be careful what you say in *here*, because you may end up out *there*.

She went easy on me for the first few sessions, even letting me borrow her copy of "The Secret" by Rhonda Byrne. I had never read any self-help books before, so I was eager to dive in and start seeing my life improve…except, the book was dog shit. I read certain sections out to my mom if I thought they sounded profound or relatable to my situation, but this adult version of "The Little Engine That Could" was not going to help me walk again.

I distinctly remember my last appointment with Molly. We had established a decent enough patient-therapist relationship that she felt comfortable being very frank in the way she spoke to me. We started the first 15 minutes or so with mom in the room, and I told her that day was my birthday, March 20th. I was wearing this striped grey turtleneck with glitter accents that mom had gotten me as a gift. Everything felt happy and hunky-dory until mom excused herself and went out to the waiting room.

I started a conversation about how we were working on figuring out a situation that allowed me to stay caught up with my schoolwork even when I wasn't able to go to my classes in person, which was most of the time, at that point. I told her that I was terrified of falling behind and I felt determined to stay on top of everything despite being sick. I wanted to go to college, after all; maybe I could get a degree in psychology, because I was becoming *so knowledgeable* about the world of mental health.

"Now Ivy," she started, "do you really think any of that will happen?" I was taken aback, but I was used to her speaking bluntly. Her tone became much darker with her affect staying the same: happy, hunky-dory.

"I think you need to quit school for a few years and focus solely on getting your life back on track." I started getting flustered as I told her that was never an option in my mind, and she looked at me like I was a kicked puppy. "Come on, now. You know that you won't be graduating with all your friends. You will never *walk* the stage. You will never progress forward in life for as long as you continue this behavior".

The dark thoughts started seeping through the cracks of my mind. I was having such a good day, too! She continued to berate me, saying things like "This is all on you. If you really wanted to have a future like you're describing, you would buckle down and work on your mental health. You are very sick, Ivy".

I dug my fingernails into my palms and started sobbing uncontrollably. "Why are you saying these things?" I whimpered, and she responded "I am just telling you the reality of the situation! You don't think you can handle the hard truth?" I felt completely, utterly worthless at that moment. I tried to remain clear-headed, but I couldn't hold back what I word-vomited next:

"I don't want to be alive anymore. I just can't do this. It hurts so bad and I want to die."

Molly grinned and leaned back in her chair. She might as well have shouted "Cut!" like she was ending a scene that she had written and directed all by herself. "That's right. Let me go get your mom, bring her back in here, and we will start the process of getting you admitted back into [Redacted hospital name]".

I went from being completely disheveled to being numb and in shock. What just happened here? My mom glided through the door with a peaceful smile on her face. She wrapped her arms around me, saying "I know, I know. It's okay. We will get you some more help".

With that, I was cast away to the nut house yet again. By then I was starting to get a "frequent flier" status, which is definitely not something you want to brag about.

<u>Chapter 11</u>

The very idea of omnipotence feels nonsensical and almost narcissistic, and I hate to admit that. I have a lot of insecurity around my lack of faith, and I feel like a major barrier for me comes from my inability to accept nuance in most things (especially those that are bigger than myself).

I loved my mother for as long as I physically could because I didn't want to accept the truth: I was a burden in her life. A mistake that she had to live with, and she made damn sure I knew that this is how she felt. Her disdain for me predated my illness, which is the most heartbreaking part for me to come to terms with.

She viewed me as an opposing force in her world that served as a penalty for her wrongdoings. Why else would God grant her someone so flawed, someone so defective, to be responsible for until the day she dies? Luckily, I don't believe in God, so I don't find myself asking similar questions. *God, why would you let me be born to a mother who didn't want me?* Shit like that doesn't have any real answers, it's just life.

There's definitely something out there in the universe; believing that there's not would be even more narcissistic and nonsensical than anything! I don't know what it is, or who "they" are, but I'm very content with not speculating. I have what I need to keep me grounded while I'm here on earth, and that just happens to be: cats. If it weren't for the existence of cats, I would without a doubt be dead.

I never had a single reservation about the people I would be leaving behind if I committed suicide, because the people closest to me made me believe I wasn't worth being missed. They would have a better life if I was gone, surely. The ones who did grieve me would at least know *why* I did it, and they would come to terms with my disappearance over time. There was only one blip in my conscience that made me think twice, a consideration that sent a searing pain throughout my body, like when you start to rip off a hangnail and you don't realize the colossal damage this will cause until your raw and bloody skin sits there mocking you.

If I were to kill myself, what would my cat Sparta think? I would be gone and he would have no way of understanding *why*. Or even worse, what if he were to find my lifeless body?

I have always been infatuated with cats, and if I believe in anything remotely spiritual, it would have to be the "Universal Cat Distribution System". It started out as a joke on TikTok, but this essentially describes a phenomenon where the universe pairs cats up with humans who need them the most. You know that corny phrase they use in rescue, "Who saved who?" I will never forget the day that I realized how my cat, Sparta, saved me.

I had just been discharged from an inpatient stay at the behavioral hospital for the third or fourth time, and I came home to an empty house; my brothers were still at school, and my dad was still at work. It was just mom and I. I made my way towards my bedroom which was in the middle of my two brothers' rooms, but when I passed the first door in the hallway I realized that my older brother's door was slightly ajar.

I peeked inside and saw Sparta sprawled out in the center of my brothers' bed like a King positioned on his throne, so I went in to say hi and let him know that I missed him while I was gone. As I sat on the edge of the bed, Sparta stood up and got onto my lap. He rolled around and forcefully headbutted my legs while I pet him for a good ten minutes or so. It was like he had missed me, and he was saying *hey, I'm glad you're back!*

Sparta never questioned the validity of my struggles or doubted that I was being truthful about being sick. He never showed me anything but unwavering, unconditional care. He was my one support system that I had left after being completely isolated by my family, and after my peers slowly left me behind. I could never inflict the pain of grieving onto him if I were to ever commit suicide. I held on for him.

I'm now an adult living away from my parents, with a person I love, and cats that we both see as family. I'll say that I have some reservations about the term "soulmate", because it carries so much weight that I don't necessarily want to unpack…however, the Universal Cat Distribution System has never failed me, and it brought me my lucky Penny.

When I graduated high school at 17 years old my mom wanted to get me a gift that was grand enough to fit the occasion, so she hopped on Craigslist and looked up "free kittens" within a 50-mile radius. We wound up bringing home a criminally small, spiky kitten who we named Shelby. Shelby was a stunning torbie who I became endlessly enamored with; when she sat in the sun, her orange accents caused the stripes in her fur to pop like fireworks.

There was no plan to get Shelby spayed because my parents are both famously anti-veterinarian. They always said that if they weren't going to spend the money to take themselves to the doctor, why the hell would they spend the money to take an animal to one? Well, one night after Shelby had just turned a year old, she ran out into the garage and refused to come inside. Mom decided to let her stay because the door was down, so it was not like she could escape. Except, we didn't realize that one of our stray cat friends who we named Richard was also in the closed garage, with Shelby, all night.

All of us gathered around a rotund Shelby about a month later and put two-and-two together. Shelby had 6 beautiful babies, and she was the best mama in the world. Richard would sit on the patio eating treats and watching his offspring through the window.

We had to keep one of the kittens, obviously, and got Shelby spayed once the babies were all weaned. The remaining kitten was my darling Dorito; an orange and white tabby who stole my heart with his silly demeanor. He looked a lot like his dad, Richard, who was a grey and white street cat with a friendly heart. Unfortunately, Richard lived a rough life outdoors and would regularly get himself into meaningless testosterone-fueled fights. He had this one wound on his side that never fully healed, and now I think I understand why, in hindsight.

When I moved out at 19, my boyfriend and I brought Shelby and Dorito with us. If Shelby wasn't caught up caring for her adult son who never moved out like the rest of her kids, she would be taking care of us. Shelby would groom my boyfriend's gelled hair for up to 30 minutes at a time, and she would lay on top of my chest or in the crook of my neck on the days that I was too weak to get out of bed. She was "Mama" more than she was "Shelby", and I am so grateful for the way she took care of me.

When Shelby developed a runny nose with persistent sneezing after getting her yearly vaccinations, we figured it was a nasty upper respiratory infection. Nothing a bit of antibiotics can't fix, right? Two months and three antibiotics later, Shelby only became sicker, and a veterinarian timidly suggested that I get her SNAP tested to check for FIV and FeLV. I had never heard of either of these conditions prior to all of this, so I'll explain it here simply:

FIV is what most people refer to as "cat AIDS". Cats with FIV have a suppressed immune system– like a person with AIDS– which makes them more prone to catching common colds and respiratory infections. These cats can live long and happy lives with proper medical intervention, when needed, and they can safely live amongst other cats. FIV is only transferred through deep bite wounds, commonly found after sexual mating takes place.

FeLV is feline leukemia, and it is considered fatal and highly contagious. Rather than having a compromised immune system, cats with feline leukemia lack the ability to fight off infection completely. Many cats have a prognosis of living 1 to 3 years after being diagnosed; something as simple as an upper respiratory infection can spiral out of control and ravage a cat's body at an alarming rate. FeLV can be transferred to other cats through close contact, meaning that FeLV+ cats must be quarantined and not share food/water bowls or litter boxes with cats that test negative.

I remember sitting next to my boyfriend amongst other people lined up for the reduced-cost vet clinic, sobbing loudly when the poor vet tech gave us the news. Shelby had tested positive for FeLV, which meant that Dorito was likely positive as well, given their familial relation. We still got Dorito tested and crossed our fingers for some sort of miracle; he was positive, as well. I started to think about Richard and that pesky wound on his side that never fully healed in the two years I knew him…

My sweet mama was only three years old when she passed. I will not describe the horrific details surrounding her last days, because watching her slowly succumb to illness was the most heartbreaking experience I have endured. She fought harder than she should have, and I wish I had let her go sooner; you should always let them go on a good day. After Shelby passed, we realized a decrease in Dorito's mood. He stopped grooming himself and was less interested in playing with his favorite toys. We figured that he must have been missing his mommy, who had taken care of him his entire life.

Dorito had also never been an "only child", so we ultimately decided that we wanted to give him a friend. This meant that the new cat would also have to be

FeLV positive. We contacted a nearby cat shelter that is held with high regard for all the amazing things they do for the surrounding communities, and they told us they had one felvie friend available for adoption.

She was an orange and white tabby with huge eyes and little socks on each paw, going by the name "Mary Ann". My boyfriend and I were directed to the very back of the "teen room", slowly navigating my wheelchair through the crowd of free-range cats up for adoption, and directed our attention towards a small closet with a chicken wire door.

Mary Ann looked up at us from her personal cat tree, and the shelter worker asked if I wanted to hold her. They placed the plump, ginger lady in my lap, and I knew there was no going back from there. My boyfriend cradled her while we were given the lore behind this chunky ball of beauty: she entered the shelter at approx. 4 months old and tested positive for FeLV, meaning she was immediately placed in quarantine. She could look out through the chicken wire door to watch the cats outside, but could never personally interact with them. Mary Ann was adopted once at about a year old, but the family returned her due to "allergies". This return happened 7 months prior to us meeting her.

We told them all about our experience with FeLV cats and they nodded along empathetically, telling us how excited they were that Mary Ann could finally find a home where she could live out her shortened life, loved and fulfilled. We decided to rename her Penelope, or "Penny" for short. My lucky, copper Penny.

Dorito was mostly indifferent toward Penny. He did not like or dislike having her around, and Penny immediately embraced her forever home. She got to look out a window for the first time in 7 months; she would growl and run away every time a car passed by. It was only a week or so later when Dorito's health plummeted, and we found ourselves in the same position as three months before when we had to say goodbye to Shelby.

We decided that euthanasia was the most humane choice, for him and ourselves. My boyfriend and I held Dorito as he took his last labored breath and finally got to rest after a long, noble battle. When we got home we were greeted by Penny, who was still in the stages of being curious about her new surroundings. My boyfriend and I sat in bed and played with Penny as we both settled into the same melancholic truth: we would have to go through this all over again in a few years when Penny inevitably gets sick.

We did not have any regrets about adopting her, as we felt that Penny was meant to be with us. In February we took Penny to get her yearly vaccinations and decided to ask for a SNAP test, just so we could be 100% sure that she did, in fact, test positive for FeLV. Before this, I emailed the shelter to ask what testing had been done while Penny was there because I assumed that they probably would have checked all the bases in order to justify keeping her in a private quarantine room for the better part of a year…I was told that they did one snap test upon intake when she was under 6 months old. A single test, which was not repeated at a later date.

At the vet, we got a SNAP and WITNESS test performed, which both displayed NEGATIVE results. We had to wait another two months before ordering an ELISA and PCR test as Penny had just been vaccinated and we didn't want that to affect the results. We needed to be completely sure before declaring that she didn't have FeLV, and these more in-depth tests would give us that peace of mind. This is the result of the IDEXX testing:
***

SEROLOGY TEST
FeLV Antigen by ELISA: NEGATIVE
MOLECULAR DIAGNOSTICS TEST
FeLV Quant RealPOR: NEGATIVE

A NEGATIVE FeLV PC result indicates that FeLV proviral DNA was not detected in the sample submitted. If Felv antigen by ELISA test recult is also negativeFelv infection is Very unlikely. Occasionally, the FeLV antigen test by ELISA may be positive in a cat with a negative FeLV PC result. This combination is most consistent with a regressive or localized FelV infection, Less commonly, the proviral DNA in the sample may be below the limit of detection, the sample may contain an uncommon strain that Is that detected by PC or the antigen test was Falsely positive.

***

Despite being elated by the news, we couldn't help but feel extremely upset at the same time. We brought Penny into a home with another positive cat, assuming that she, herself, was positive. Even though Dorito was only around Penny for about a week before he died, the fact that he could have transmitted this infection to Penny during that time is mortifying. The part that I just cannot get over is the fact that Penny was needlessly in quarantine for so, so long. She could look out and see other cats, but never interact with them. She was needlessly isolated and neglected by people who should have known better.

I urge everyone to do their research and get proper confirmation when a cat tests positive for FeLV. In a PDF from the idexx website that addresses common questions regarding the SNAP test and how they should be interpreted, it states "kittens tested before 6 months of age that are positive should be retested at 60-day intervals. If tests performed after 6 months of age are still confirmed positive, these kittens should be considered infected". It's also extremely important to remember that you are only interpreting the test after exactly 10 minutes, because "after 10 minutes, color development may occur that is not related to the sample."

Once a cat has been re-SNAP tested multiple times, I would still advise looking into an ELISA and PCR test. These two tests cost me around $230 and I believe this investment would be more than worth it to ensure that no other cat has to go through what Penny did.

Penny may just be a cat, but she knows what I went through. She may not even remember her days in the shelter, and she might have even enjoyed having her own space! But she was treated differently, and she had to spend all of kitten-hood being hidden away due to a deadly virus that she didn't even have. What happened to me is unacceptable, but I am now at least able to share my story. Penny cannot vouch for herself or her personal experiences, however, So I will always be her #1 advocate. I will advocate for *all* cats with FeLV and spread awareness about the importance of following proper testing protocols. Penny takes care of me in a different way than Shelby did; less of a motherly presence, and more like a best friend.

Thank you, Universe, for giving me my Penny.

Chapter 12

My mom has a nasty habit of saying the cruelest, most traumatizing things she can think of when she gets angry. Her words are like rusty daggers that she would plunge into our most vulnerable parts, only so she could chastise us later on when we wound up with tetanus. She wanted to do a maximal amount of damage in the moment; it baffled my mother when we would bring up some of the things she said to us years later, because we weren't supposed to hold onto those words. If she was over it, we should've been, too.

Years after we found out that I didn't actually have Conversion Disorder, she would tell me how she only said what she did because she figured I would eventually get tired of the verbal abuse and stop faking everything. She tells me that she never *really* meant it when she threatened and berated me, she did because she thought it would help better me as a person.

"As soon as you turn 18," mom growled between drags of a cigarette, "you're out of my house. I will kick your ass to the curb whether or not you can walk".

Funnily enough, when I moved out at 19, she nearly disowned me for taking my monthly SSI checks with me.

"Either that, or I will have to go into debt to put you in a nursing home. I'll probably lose my house and we will end up on the street, while you are livin' it up in some fucking assisted living facility". Mom really liked to place the burden of our entire family and the house we lived in on my shoulders, as if we were constantly one bad day away from setting up camp on a dirty bus bench.

She told me stories about how bad the living conditions are in nursing homes, which she would know, because she's worked in a few of them. Maybe I would get lucky and have a CNA that would take enough pity on me to change my diaper, but I would more than likely be left to marinate in my own shit and piss as pressure sores the size of my fist formed on my backside. I also needed to take into account that I was "young and cute", so the male workers would eventually take advantage of that. Nobody would be there to save me, and *nobody would ever believe me* if I said something.

She claims that she only said these things because she thought it would scare me straight.

Impromptu interventions were usually conducted by mom alone because she preferred to ride solo. However, in an attempt to pack a greater punch, she would occasionally involve my brothers or father. I can vividly recall the day she called us all into the living room so that she could instruct [older brother], [younger brother], and dad to sit on the couch as I stood facing them about 10 feet away. My knuckles turned white as I gripped the handles on my walker, and my knees buckled inwards.

Mom stood perpendicular to me and declared the floor to be open for anyone who had anything they wanted to say to me…and she was met with silence. I braced myself for impact, but nobody said a word. Mom started to get agitated and began ordering them to speak, one by one.

First was dad, who told me that he loved me very much, but he wasn't sure what I needed from him in order to be happy. He just wanted me to get better.

Then my younger brother, who whimpered and asked me why I hated my family as a whole. He regurgitated everything mom had been feeding him over the years; why do you want us to get taken away by CPS? Why do you want us to become homeless? Why do you want to hurt us?

My older brother got his turn last, but he gruffly refused. He simply sat and stared right past me looking dejected and disgusted. My older brother was the first person I ever idolized, and he hated my fucking guts.

That was all pretty good, but mom wanted to wrap up this gift with a nice, shiny ribbon. "Pull your pants down, now" she commanded. I looked over at her with my mouth agape, like, *what?* My immediate concern was over my brothers and father seeing me in my underwear. She barked at me that I didn't have a choice and that my shirt would cover me enough. I shamefully lowered my jeans until they were around my knees, and I could feel the air around me solidifying. I couldn't seem to breathe as everyone examined my bruised, slashed-up thighs.

"See what she does? See what she's willing to do for attention?" Mom was like a dog proudly presenting a mangled squirrel carcass to its' horrified owners.

After the family was allowed to disband, I sat by myself on the tattered green couch and disassociated. I knew that my family hated me, but mom wanted to be sure I didn't forget. She wanted to be sure they remained on the right side of history, which meant keeping me isolated and thoroughly despised. Dad was out in the garage either drinking or smoking weed, my brothers were in their rooms, and mom had just gotten out of the shower when she called me back to the master bedroom where she could confront me alone.

I stood in the doorway feeling physically exhausted from the walk to get to the other end of the house, and she stood on the other side of the room as she violently brushed through her wet curls. I couldn't imagine how she could make me feel any worse at that point, but mom is a master of her trade.

"You know, Ivy…I didn't sign up for this. You were born *healthy*. I gave birth to a *perfect* daughter".

She reminded me of this quite often in an attempt to make me feel guilty for being sick. Remember: she will always be the biggest victim. She will always take first place in the trauma Olympics. I don't want to come across as callous or unempathetic, because I do believe that my parents had to grieve the "normal" child they once had.

She slowly walked towards me as she continued, saying "I never wanted to have a sick kid. I decided before any of you were born that I was not equipped to take care of a disabled child, so I would not allow myself to have one. If the doctor would have told me that you would end up like this…I would have gotten an abortion".

Ouch, but, okay. This is still valid to me; most people aren't willing to admit that they would not knowingly give birth to a disabled baby that would need specialized care for at least some portion of its life. A lot of people are afraid to say these things out loud for fear of being viewed as heartless monsters, but I can absolutely see why someone would feel this way. I'm willing to give mom credit where credit seems due, however…nothing will ever make up for what she said to me next.

"You need to stop looking for alternative answers to explain all of this. Conversion Disorder is your best bet, because it means that you will not be permanently disabled. You don't *want* to be sick, like, for real!" It pissed me off every time she framed the situation as if I *wanted* things to be this way.

"If the doctors were to find out that you have one of those diseases you always bring up, like MS or ALS, we would have to send you away. I am not strong enough to take care of a disabled child for the rest of my life. I would end up committing suicide to escape a reality like that, because I just don't want it!" I just stood in front of her feeling numb and defeated.

She put on her best pair of puppy dog eyes and spoke in a whisper, pleading "So please…stop fighting this diagnosis. We want you to have Conversion Disorder. We want you to get better".

There you go, folks. You know that nagging feeling in the pit of your stomach that you've had on the back burner, making you want to say that I need to be less harsh on my parents because they are clearly victims, too? My mother and father want people to believe they were scared, vulnerable parents who got taken advantage of by corrupt doctors that only had their best interests in mind.

My parents are not stupid. My parents were not ignorant. My parents were not kept "in the dark". They knew that something was seriously wrong with me, and they refused to face it for as long as they possibly could. *See no evil, hear no evil, speak no evil.* My parents are vile people who never truly loved me because of things I can't control. I constantly grieve the mom and dad that I needed but never had. I constantly miss my siblings who were turned against me to further a malevolent agenda written by my own mother.

The worst part about my mother's unrepentant threats to send me away is the fact that I knew she would never actually follow through. Mom could never handle the shame and embarrassment of sending one of her children to a care facility because she, herself, couldn't provide them the care they needed. She would have kept me around for as long as she or I lived and made sure that I spent every waking moment enthralled with guilt over what a burden I was to her. She would remind me of everything I stole from her, as if she had anything to take.

Chapter 13

By the time I was 15 years old, I had ended up wheelchair-bound. We found a small charter high school that was right down the road from where my father worked, and we were delighted to find out that my aunt (my father's sister) was the guidance counselor on campus. The entire school was so small that it was probably less than a tenth the size of *[redacted Highschool]*.

They didn't have AP classes or extracurricular courses; the school day went from 8 AM to 12 PM, and students were given a chance at an "accelerated" path toward graduating. It was a get in and get out as quick as possible sort of operation for kids who had trouble staying on track at "regular" high schools. I was heartbroken by the thought of not having the traditional high school experience I had always dreamed of, but this seemed like my best shot at getting my diploma before I was 25.

When I see people with walkers or, god forbid, someone in a wheelchair, my sympathy response is automatically triggered. What a shame, to be disabled...*the cripple thought.* It's truly bizarre how disconnected I still am from my own body all these years later. Sometimes I randomly "remember" that I can't walk, my legs don't work, and I get a little bummed out. I wasn't in an accident that changed my life in a flash. I had to slowly succumb to disability during my most influential years as a developing teenager, without a support system to soften the blow.

We showed up for my interview/orientation for the school and got greeted by a woman with a comforting southern drawl who directed us towards an empty classroom, which was about 200 feet away. I stared down the short hallway as my knees were already buckling when I heard a cheerful voice telling me "Don't worry, take your time!" By the time I sat down again, I was too exhausted to remember any of the questions I had prepared for this meeting. I just wanted to go home and sleep.

When everything was said and done and we completed my registration, I slowly lifted myself up out of the hard, plastic chair. My arms trembled and I bit down on my lower lip as I turned towards the exit, but as soon as I cleared the doorway, I collapsed. Mom gasped hysterically while every nearby staff member rushed over to help me stand back up again. They grabbed me a chair to sit in while mom pulled the car up to the front of the building, and I basked in the embarrassment of being escorted out by my future principal and Economics teacher.

This was also around the time that I had to learn how to self-cath. While my kidneys were holding up fine, my bladder was only emptying about twenty percent of the way when it was completely full. This meant frequent bathroom trips and lots of smaller accidents in between, because a poise pad can only hold so much dribble. Having all that old urine sitting around caused irritation to the lining of my bladder and, you guessed it, recurring urinary tract infections.

I remember sitting on the toilet staring down at my vagina in a handheld mirror, completely listless, as mom stood outside the door in case I caved and decided to ask for help. If there are trained nurses out there who can't get a catheter into their female patients, how the hell was I supposed to get one in myself?

I was quickly becoming very…well, disabled. I couldn't walk anymore, and I couldn't even piss properly without sticking a straw up my urethra. I had to sit on a bench when I showered. I had to wear depends. I had to go to a shitty charter school that was made for delinquent kids who hated going to school.

Even though we were still running with the whole "Conversion Disorder" plot, I was undeniably miserable. I was getting sicker, and it was nearly impossible to claim that I was manufacturing my illness as a means of garnering attention and sympathy. Mom knew that things were heading down a dark road, so she hesitantly started to lean into advocacy, as opposed to denying that anything was *actually* wrong with me.

I sat quietly and watched as my primary care physician quickly typed away, updating my chart accordingly. I was there for my yearly checkup and I let mom do all the talking, as I had been trained. Except this time, I could sense my mother's *fear*. Her voice quivered a little as she stated,

"You know, we have been seeing Dr. E every three months for the last three years, and she has refused to do any sort of follow-up testing. She did one follow-up MRI of Ivy's spine, and that's it."

The doctor looked at me with an expression that I now understand was likely a mix of anticipation and guilt, but at the time, we thought she was just as worried about my declining health as we were. She knew that something was up, and she was realizing that *we knew*, as well.

"Dr. E really isn't going to appreciate this…she is the one who is supposed to handle your neurology related care."

I'm sure I scoffed or expressed some sort of annoyance before the doctor continued to say "But, you are right, I think Ivy is due for another MRI. I am going to order a scan of her brain this time." The doctor strained as she attempted to maintain a chipper tone. We were satisfied with this and left the clinic that day with a scheduled brain MRI. These are the results of the spine MRI scans that Dr. E ordered a year prior to this appointment (one year after she diagnosed me with Conversion Disorder):

***

MRI THORACIC SPINE W WO CONTRAST
Collected on July 9, 2015 3:42 PM

Impression: 1. There is a focal area of increased T2 signal in the spinal cord and at approximately the level of the T7 vertebral body. This has the appearance of a spinal cord infarct. However, this cannot be confirmed on other sequences and may represent artifact.

Exam: MRI thoracic spine without and with contrast.

History: Back pain.

Findings: MRI of the thoracic spine was performed in the axial and sagittal planes using T1 and T2 weighted sequences. These images are supplemented by coronal T2 weighted sequences. The vertebral body height, marrow signal, and alignment is normal. The intervertebral discs are normal. No spinal canal stenosis is noted. There is no abnormal enhancement after intravenous contrast infusion. There is increased T2 signal in the center of the cord on series 1301/image 25. However, this area cannot be confirmed on other sequences and may represent artifact. A spinal cord infarct can have this appearance.

MRI LUMBAR SPINE W WO CONTRAST
Collected on July 9, 2015 3:37 PM

Impression: 1. Normal MRI of the lumbar spine.
Exam: MRI lumbar spine without and with contrast.
Clinical history: Back pain.
Findings: MRI of the lumbosacral spine was performed in the axial and sagittal planes using T1 and T2-weighted sequences. These images are supplemented by coronal T2-weighted sequences. 12.2 mL of Magnevist was administered and the T1-weighted sequences were repeated. The vertebral body height, marrow signal, and alignment normal. The

intervertebral discs are normal. The conus medullaris is located at the superior endplate of the L1 vertebral body and is of normal signal. There is no evidence of a fatty filum terminale. There is no abnormal enhancement after intravenous contrast infusion.

***

My next appointment with Dr. E was not long after this. Mom must have had a small fire lit under her ass because her confidence was growing. "You know," mom said in a matter-of-fact tone, "we got the PCP to order some further testing for Ivy. I think it's a good idea, so we can make sure we aren't missing anything." Dr. E kept her eyes glued to her computer screen as she spoke slowly, struggling to hide her distaste.

"Yes, well, that's very nice. I do wish she would have consulted with me first before ordering it, though!" Dr. E said in an uppity, agitated tone.

I was coasting off of mom's energy and bravely added "I know you always tell me that you have tested me for 'every possibility under the sun', but that just isn't true." Dr. E turned towards me in an ominous fashion.

"Where are you getting that idea from?" Dr. E asked in an infantilizing tone.

"Well, what about a lumbar puncture? We never did that. I read that you need a lumbar puncture to diagnose MS." I stated.

The doctor shook her head and smiled as if I had just pooped my pants and asked for more apple juice in my sippy cup.

"I'm sure you also read that a lumbar puncture is a very *dangerous* procedure! I just can't see why we would need to do that to you" she cooed.

I stood my ground (well…sat?) and pushed further. I wasn't exactly keen on the thought of a 10-foot needle being pushed into my spine, but I would do virtually anything for some answers at this point.

"Okay, fine. What else can we try, then? What tests have we not done yet?"

I stared daggers through her hardened demeanor, before Dr. E finally spoke, saying,

"Ah, well…I guess we could do an EMG. However, you'll have to travel *all the way* to San Antonio to get one done. That's the closest place available for this sort of specialized testing."

I glanced back at mom nervously, because I knew that a 3 hour drive for a single medical test was definitely not ideal.

Mom wrung her hands together while she responded, "Okay, sure. We can do that". Dr. E flung her hands up as if to say *okay, you got me!* We sat silently as she timidly typed in the order, before Dr. E said "I think I'll also throw in an an audiogram, because why not?" Mom and I both gave each other a look that communicated our mutual understanding; Dr. E wanted to make us look stupid by ordering stupid tests that we knew would come back normal.

Sure enough, I passed the test with no evidence of hearing loss…though, there's no record that I completed the test at all. In MyChart, I can see **"*AUDIOGRAM*, Collected on May 24, 2016 11:18 AM",** but the results area was left completely blank.

<u>Chapter 14</u>

What is an EMG? According to John Hopkins Medicine,

"Electromyography (EMG) measures muscle response or electrical activity in response to a nerve's stimulation of the muscle. The test is used to help detect neuromuscular abnormalities. During the test, one or more small needles (also called electrodes) are inserted through the skin into the muscle."

Okay, but…what does that really mean? I was about to find out.

Up until that point, I had never really traveled anywhere outside my city. We never visited relatives in other states or took family vacations, so I was excited to see San Antonio! I was surprised by the amount of cows and open farmland we drove past, and I was shocked by the number of homeless individuals in the area surrounding our destination, the hospital. We wound up going into the wrong building at first, making us late for our appointment with Dr. T, another pediatric neurologist, and colleague of Dr. E.

Mom was frantic by the time we found the right place to check-in, and we were almost immediately ushered away to a room by Dr. T himself. He was older and had crow's feet around his eyes when he smiled, which made me ease up slightly. He tugged at his surgical cap as my parents and I settled in, asking "How was the drive here? I heard y'all had a long journey".

"It wasn't so bad! I'm just glad to finally be here and getting this done", mom said, staying overly cordial. Dr. T stayed quiet while I sat on the table with a sheet over my exposed legs. I watched nervously as he set up the testing equipment and explained to me what he was about to do.

"You see this? It's actually a wire, a *teeny tiny* wire. There will be no needles involved, just my little wires". Dr. T said with a phony grin on his face. I glanced over at dad as he was nervously shifting in his seat.

"What I'm going to do is stick the wires into your skin and test different muscles in your legs by sending small electrical currents through the wires. When I ask you to contract those muscles, it will show me how they respond to the electricity. Not too hard, right?" He recited this speech swiftly, without breaking eye contact.

When you are being treated as a pediatric patient, the doctor will typically do what they can to make you feel calm and less afraid. I wasn't exactly feeling cool and collected, but dad looked as though he was about to blow chunks. Mom noticed his restlessness and spoke to him in a hushed tone, saying "Stop it, you will be fine. You can go 45 minutes without a fucking cigarette". Dad nodded and clutched his chest, responding "I know, I know".

I've never given birth or had kidney stones, and most people online will tell you that the EMG study is only mildly uncomfortable. Yet, I will still confidently state that my EMG was the most excruciating, horrific pain I have ever been through. I have been terrified of needles for as long as I can remember. My phobia has subdued with age, but I was only 16 years old at the time and I was still tentative about everything happening around me.

The neurologist, who I had only just met, attempted to make small talk as he placed little stickers in various spots on my legs. "So, how long have you been in the wheelchair? You can't walk at all?" He inquired casually.

"Well, it's been about…" he peeled up one of the stickers along with a dozen leg hairs while I was in the middle of my sentence, causing me to yelp. "Sorry, I accidentally placed it in the wrong spot," the doctor said, smiling sheepishly. These sticky electrodes are the same thing you would deal with when using a tens unit…*no biggie,* I thought, *I have done this before.*

First I felt the sticker electrodes going off. "Ouch. Yeah, okay, that doesn't feel…good?" I spoke timidly. "Yeah, some slight discomfort is to be expected," said the doctor with a wave of his hand. *Slight discomfort.* Dr. T glanced up at me, asking "Are you sure you don't want another pillow before we start?" I shook my head no. "Alright, then. There's going to be a slight pinch" he stated.

Cue the sobs. I must have screamed so loud that it scared the doctors beside manner away, sending it flying out the window. "You need to calm down! You need to breathe, stop it!" He pleaded, and I pleaded back, repeating "I can't do this, please stop".

Mom stood up and came over to pet my head while dad stayed glued to his chair. Mom told me that it would be okay and that I could do this, but it was becoming increasingly clear that dad could *not*. I watched my father pull a bandanna out of his pocket and wipe his forehead feverishly, saying "I'm sorry, I just get nervous around needles. It's so hard to see her in pain like this". The doctor looked at us with his mouth slightly agape, as if he was in a mockumentary and they were about to comedically zoom in on his dumbfounded face.

"Okay, this is the hard part", the doctor spoke slowly as if he thought I might get up and run away. I sniffled and listened intently.

"I'm going to send an electrical current through the wire which will make your muscles contract involuntarily. You'll also feel electric pulses from the stickers, okay? When I tell you to contract a specific muscle, you need to tense up as hard as you can". I had already told him that I was afraid I wouldn't be able to do this part because my legs *didn't work*. I still needed to at least try; if my muscles were deteriorating, this test would show it.

The last legal execution via electric chair without an *alternative* method offered took place in the year 2002. After multiple instances where individuals had been unnecessarily electrocuted multiple times before finally dying, the courts ruled this method of execution to be "cruel and unusual punishment". Nothing could have prepared me for the internal spark show that was about to light up the muscle fibers in my spaghetti noodle legs. Speaking of spaghetti, have you ever accidentally touched the edge of a hot pot while cooking a meal on the stove? In just a fraction of a second, you can end up with an angry burn that mocks you for weeks to come as it heals slowly.

The electricity spread like ripples in a pond that were set off by a burning hot coal. I saw flashes of light that were only visible to me as I shrieked uncontrollably. I let go of my mother's hand and dug my nails into my palms while I berated the neurologist.

"Why does it hurt so bad? What are you doing?!" I demanded answers from the doctor who was gradually becoming more aggravated, and we had only just started. He raised up out of his stool and stared me down, speaking sternly, saying:

"You are overreacting in a MAJOR way. I have done this test on myself so I can know personally what my patients have to endure, and I know for a *fact* that this doesn't hurt *that* bad."

Mom was visibly taken aback as if she had never seen a doctor accuse me of fabricating my pain before, and dad put his pale face into his sweaty palms.

"Do you want to continue? If you can't control yourself, I have to stop." Dr. T threatened. I knew that I had to complete the test because I was clinging to the possibility that they would finally find something wrong with me.

"I'm sorry, I can do it. It just hurts so, so bad." I spoke between sharp gasps for air. "I'm going to cry, I have to be able to cry".

He nodded curtly and continued the study. I wailed like a grieving widow after each burst of electricity and spent the pauses in between hyperventilating. I would have kicked the doctor square in his smug fucking face if I had the ability to do so. When he told me to tense up, I did, but I had no idea if anything was actually registering. Even though my lower half was generally rendered useless, my spasming limbs made rips in the parchment paper covering the bed underneath me.

Around halfway through the melodrama of watching me get electrocuted, my father finally stood up…not for me, but, to leave the room before he passed out. He tried to ward mom off with profuse apologies but she still followed him out after asking the doctor for a 5 minute break. I appreciated the intermission, but I knew that dad was about to have a royal ass chewing on the drive back home.

By the time the EMG was finished, I felt like the doctor was playing a cruel practical joke when he announced "That's it, we're done with the test. I need to review the results now". His face contorted as he evaluated the random assortment of squiggly lines on the screen in front of him. I twiddled my thumbs impatiently for what felt like decades when the doctor finally let out a strained sigh and reported "Well, here's the thing. There's good news and bad news here".

I felt a lump forming in my throat while my parents leaned in slowly, carefully.

"You see, here's the *good* news," Dr. T began. "The test shows that Ivy's muscles are healthy and intact; no deterioration or atrophy is noted. However…" my stomach dropped slightly. *How could my muscles be perfectly fine if I can't walk?*

The doctor cleared his throat nervously before saying "Ivy has neuropathy. Small fiber neuropathy, to be exact. This leads me to believe that there is something going on internally that is preventing her nerves from sending proper communications to the muscles, which is why she can't seem to use them".

Well…fuck! Mom and dad were distraught, and I was simply in disbelief. The doctor seemed listless as he rattled off a few conditions and diseases that can cause this form of neuropathy before telling us that we would be best off consulting with the neurologist in charge of my care: Dr. E. We left that day with more questions than ever before, and without any meaningful answers in sight. The atmosphere on the car ride home was tense, with an unsettling undertone of dread that emanated from my parents.

I felt residual shocks throughout my body for months to follow; the sensation was randomized and unrelenting. Nothing made the pain better or worse, so I had to live with surprise electrical attacks for a good chunk of time, on top of searing neuropathy pain, which I finally had a label for.

I would gladly share the report of my EMG results if I could…on paper, there's no record of this test ever happening. I searched the deepest depths of my MyChart and scoured the physical copies of my medical records; it's almost as though these results were buried and deleted from existence.

<u>Chapter 15</u>

Mom always told me that I saw things through rose-colored glasses. I would sit and watch her dig through her closet, trying to find the perfect outfit to wear for a family function that was full of people she dreaded seeing, and I'd tell her how pretty she would look *no matter what.* She'd smile, unenthused, and say "Of course *you* think that, sweetie. Because I'm your mom!"

There was a major shift in the dynamic between mom and I after the EMG. She spoke to me in a softer, more heedful fashion, like I was fine China that might crack if she wasn't careful. Two days after the test was performed, there was a call from a very disgruntled Dr. E.

Mom put the phone on speaker and motioned for me to stay quiet. "So," said the doctor, "I was looking at the results of Ivy's EMG". Her tone was prudent and laced with bitterness. My mom chirped back, "Yes! Can you believe it?" Dr. E scoffed harshly.

"I am just as surprised as you are, Mrs. Babbitt…don't you worry". The doctor's voice raised a couple of octaves, and she proclaimed "I will find out how she did it!"

Sorry…*what?*

Mom's face dropped and we both looked at each other in confusion. "I am going to figure out how she managed to manipulate the test into showing these results! I cannot believe she has done this!" Dr. E blurted out. I watched my mother's jaw drop, which was very validating. We were *both* speechless at this moment.

Mom must have been able to hear the uneasiness in the doctor's voice and knew that it would be unwise to start an argument over the phone with no credible witnesses, so she confirmed our upcoming appointment and left things on a seemingly positive note. She stared blankly at the wall while muttering "What the hell is going on right now?"

She then sat in front of her computer and asked me "What was the name of that thing you think you have?" Of all the possibilities to explain my symptoms, MS seemed to make the most sense, so I had brought it up quite a few times. She read out loud as she typed,

"Symptoms…of….multiple…how do you spell sclerosis?"

I watched as she practically inverted like a terrified turtle while reading a play-by-play of what I had been going through for the past 6 years. She chuckled nervously and favorited one of the pages, saying "Well, who knows, maybe you do have something like that".

I desperately wanted to gloat and say *no shit, you stupid motherfucker,* but I couldn't. Instead, I sheepishly reminded her that she needed to schedule an optometrist appointment for me. My vision was becoming increasingly unreliable, and I was due for some cute new frames. She snapped out of her daze and choked out "Oh, you're right. Let me look up someone who will take your insurance". And thus, we came across Dr. D.

The spark that ended up setting off an explosive chain reaction of exposing the truth wound up being a routine optometrist visit. You know how they say that the eyes are the window to the soul? It turns out that they are also a bit of a window to the *brain.* I transferred over to the squeaky rubber exam chair which was connected to the ophthalmoscope, and mom parked my wheelchair in the back corner of the room.

While we waited in silence for the doctor, I studied the letters on the seeing-eye chart. *I'm definitely going to need a stronger prescription,* I thought.

Dr. D was a friendly woman who introduced herself to mom and I before taking a moment to glance at my chart one more time. "So, I'm seeing that you listed 'Conversion Disorder' under her pre-existing medical conditions?"

Mom sat slumped over in her chair and responded "Uh, yeah. She can't walk", seeming unamused. The doctor narrowed her eyes before scanning me from top to bottom, from my anxious brows to my deadened toes.

"Huh. Well, okay! Let's take a look at your eyes, then" she finally asserted.

I started feeling nervous as I read off the letters and symbols on the eye chart, which made mom laugh and say "This isn't some kind of test, honey. It's okay if you get some wrong!" The doctor handed me a small plastic paddle, saying "Use this to cover up your left eye for me," to which I obliged. I was taken aback by how blurry my world became in an instant, and I stuttered through a couple of the top rows before Dr. D told me I had done enough.

I took the dilation drops like a champ and did my best to choose between *lens one, or lens two? Lens two, or lens three?* The doctor paused like she was trying to stifle a sneeze, and glanced back at my sad, empty wheelchair. "Why are you in a wheelchair, again?" she asked in a dubious tone. Mom let out a displeased sigh, so I went ahead and answered,

"They say that the Conversion Disorder is what causes me to not be able to walk. I have really bad anxiety…I guess".

"Oh, I see…" the doctor spoke softly as she pondered what she was about to say next. I started to pick at my cuticles nervously as I prepared myself to be lectured by yet another doctor about how I was obviously fine and allowing myself to waste away in that *darn* chair. She turned her attention back to staring at me through the scope.

Doctor: So, just out of curiosity, has anyone ever mentioned the white spot you have on your optic nerve?

Me: Uh, no, I don't think so?

Mom: No one has ever mentioned that to us before, no.

Me: Why, is that something bad?

Doctor: Well, it *can* be, but it might also be nothing…it's the sort of thing that you typically see in patients who have chronic conditions, like, I don't know…MS, for example.

Mom immediately sat up and gripped her purse, blurting out "Are you fucking kidding me?" I laughed cautiously before mom composed herself, saying "Sorry, sorry, I shouldn't have cursed like that". The doctor's affect became worried and skeptical as she studied our reactions.

"Well, " Dr. D started, "this is really something I would like a specialist to look at, we don't have the equipment here that is needed to get a better look at the optic nerves and whatnot".

I looked over at the bullets of sweat forming on mom's forehead and started zoning out while the doctor continued to speak. "I'm going to put in an emergency referral for you to see an ophthalmologist" she stated. We ended up getting an appointment with an ophthalmology firm *two days later*. I don't want to brag or anything, but, such speed in booking is virtually unheard of with most specialists.

I didn't know it at the time, but now I understand that I must have been in pretty bad shape to create such urgency. The alarm bells had been ringing since the very beginning, but people were only just now able to hear them going off.

Chapter 16

We pulled up to a building with rounded rectangular windows and an overall vintage feel. I focused on taking evenly-paced breaths as we rode up to the second floor in an elevator that smelt like burning rubber and old pennies.

The waiting area was jam-packed with senior citizens which made me feel a tad self-conscious, until I spotted a young couple sitting with an infant wrapped up in a blanket. There was a nurse telling them that the drops should start to kick in soon, and the mother looked down at the baby in her arms who was whimpering quietly, while the father cooed "I know, I know. The doctor is going to see you very soon". *Well, at least I'm not the youngest patient here,* I thought.

Mom began filling out the new patient paperwork as she had done so many times before, but she stopped and stared uncomfortably only a few pages in. The sheet in front of her inquired about symptoms and chief concerns related to the patient's vision.

"Um…maybe you should fill this part out", she said, handing me the pen and clipboard.

I checked boxes next to various items such as *blurred vision, floaters, seeing bright flashes of light, eye fatigue.* Mom scanned over my answers and frowned. "You know, I can fill out the rest if you want me to", I offered. I was 16 years old at this point, so surely I could fill out some basic questionnaires, right? Mom shook her head no and quickly grabbed the clipboard from me like an animal that was resource guarding its dinner.

Before anything else, I was taken back to a room by that same familiar nurse and given a handful of different drops. One of the drops was yellow like popcorn butter and made my eyeballs feel like someone had rolled them around on a paper towel before placing them back in my skull. I watched the fish tank in the middle of the waiting room become more and more blurry until the doctor finally called my name. There was Dr. C, who was the main provider, and Dr. W, who was a resident in training. My recollection of events isn't too good, but I do remember Dr. W taking the reins, for the most part.

He started by getting a good look at my eyes using various hand-held lenses and a headlamp. I looked up, down, left, and right, exactly like that one time at my neurology appointment where Dr. E took inexplicable interest in my eyes. He would say things out loud for the nurse to jot down, and none of it made any sense to me, but none of it *sounded* particularly good.

One of the tests they had me do was a visual field study. Basically, you look through what feels like a large set of plastic goggles and play a little video game where you press a button every time you see the blinking dots on the screen move; the catch is that you can only look directly ahead. If your eyes move in any other direction the machine will sense this and pause the test. This helps check your peripheral vision and if it is being hindered at all.

They took dozens of pictures of my eyes that day, but one set of photographs had to be obtained by completing a "fluorescein angiogram". This involved injecting a contrast dye through an IV before taking pictures of my retina, checking for abnormal blood vessels. Dr. W warned me that the dye tends to make people feel extremely nauseous, but once it was injected I needed to get in front of the machine right away to take the pictures.

He nudged the trashcan in my direction in case I thought I was going to throw up, and I laughed because it seemed so silly.

It turns out that I was overly confident in my gut and almost immediately felt a tsunami of nausea crashing down on me. I started to panic because it truly seemed like I was about to vomit all over the tiny office, and Dr. W scrambled to hand me a couple of alcohol wipes, instructing me to hold them up to my nose."The smell of the alcohol will help with feeling sick, I promise," he told me as I composed myself.

I did not upchuck that day, but I did have some very orange pee for the rest of the day as the contrast dye left my system. After almost two hours of non-stop tests, we were finally sent back to the waiting room while they looked over all of my results. I closed my tired eyes and leaned my head back, daydreaming about the incredible nap I was about to take when I got home. It took quite a while until Dr. W peered around the corner and called my name again, quietly this time. Mom quickly pushed me over to the somber doctor who stayed silent on our way back to a private office.

Dr. W was a very fair-skinned man of Polish descent, and in that moment he surpassed the description of "white as a ghost". I had never seen someone look at me with such intense dread. He fumbled with a folder of all my imaging done that day before stuttering out the same exact question that everyone seemed to be asking me around this time:

"Ivy, tell me again…why is it that you are in a wheelchair? Why can't you walk?"

I gave him the same spiel and explained that I had been told there was nothing wrong with me, physically, and I was disabled due to a severe case of "anxiety".

There are 3 main issues that they found that day:

1. Uveitis. There were free-floating cells inside the vitreous of my eyes, which was likely a result of…

2. Macular edema. Blood vessels were leaking into the macula, which is part of the retina, causing this area to swell. ME can cause blurry vision and progressive vision loss. The results of my visual field test showed that the damage to my retinas was affecting my peripheral vision.

3. Lastly, I had something called gliosis. Dr. W explained this to me using an analogy, saying "Imagine what happens when you wrap a rubber band around your finger; it cuts off the blood circulation. Cells are cutting off the blood circulation to your optic nerves like small rubber bands".

After allowing us a moment to digest this gigantic dump of foreign information, Dr. W leaned in and spoke with a quiver in his voice, telling us "This is incredibly serious. Your daughter is sick, and I am worried that she might end up with permanent vision loss if you do not urgently seek out a second opinion".

The doctor told us about one of his colleagues who worked at a children's hospital 4 hours away from us; a neurology resident named Dr. G. "You need to get out of [this city] and establish a new network of medical providers. I am shocked that this has gone on for so long" Dr. W said with a disgusted scowl. "I also recommend you obtain copies of *all* of her medical records, from birth to present day. I have a feeling you will find a lot of information in them that has been withheld" he advised.

I looked over at mom and watched as her little imaginary bubble of safety quickly deflated, leaving her completely exposed to a nightmarish reality that she never wanted to face. I also took a moment to survey all 4 corners of the small room looking for hidden cameras, as if someone was about to bust down the door and tell me that this whole thing was an elaborate prank. I did not feel afraid from the grim prognosis, and I did not feel joy for the fact that the truth was finally becoming apparent. I felt no emotions at all. I did not know how I was *allowed* to feel.

As mom and I shuffled over to the receptionist in charge of checking people out, Dr. W stopped us and handed me a thin piece of transparent black plastic, telling me "You can put these behind your glasses, they'll block out the sunlight while the dilation drops wear off". I fastened my snazzy new shades and stared at the ground while mom and Dr. W made a call to Dr.

G's office. We ended up getting an appointment scheduled for two and a half months later, which gave us plenty of time to gather my records and get everything in order with the insurance.

After loading my wheelchair into the trunk, mom sat and gripped the steering wheel while watching the handicapped parking sign in front of us, as if the little person on it was about to stand up out of their chair and say *just kidding, I'm not disabled!* She grimaced and shifted in her seat uncomfortably before turning to me slowly, asking

"So, uh…wanna get some McDonalds on the way home?"

<u>Chapter 17</u>

A younger version of myself saw immense glamor in being a sick kid; spoken like a true *regular* kid. I grew up incredibly normal and relatively healthy. I remember going to the children's hospital for routine checkups and whatnot, and I would ask "Mom, can we go to the playground after the doctor's appointment?" Mom would shake her head and smile warmly at silly little me, responding, "No, honey. That's there for the kids with cancer and stuff". Well, I don't have cancer, but I definitely have…stuff.

I sure wished I had cancer, though! I would see the St. Jude commercials with bald children getting gifted iPads, puppies, and race cars, and think to myself: *could they be any more lucky? I wish I was on TV!* It never occurred to me that these kids were facing literal mortality, and no amount of flashy presents or celebrity cameos would make the poison being injected into their veins any less painful. I was blissfully ignorant for so long.

I felt very uneasy about the way everyone's attitude toward me began to shift. My father was more outwardly affectionate towards me now that mom was no longer gatekeeping the ability to interact with me in any positive capacity. My younger brother constantly asked me if I needed any favors or if he could do anything to help me, and my older brother started to buy me miscellaneous gifts like T-shirts and fast food. It pissed me the fuck off to see all of them so wracked with guilt because they should have believed me from the very beginning. My mother should have advocated for me. My father should have protected me. My siblings should have loved me enough to see that I wasn't lying to them.

I struggle with a very latent form of disassociation; it doesn't hit me like a quirky Scrubs-style daydream, but it definitely has the ability to stop me in my tracks. I never got to properly grieve my abled body because I was constantly told that I was fine and I would be back to normal in no time. I was forced into a brainwashed state of attempting to heal as a form of survival, because my inevitable deterioration was treated as if it was a form of disobedience.

Watching videos of my past self fills me with a unique mixture of rage and sorrow; not because I feel sorry for me, but because I feel sorry for *her*. I am horrified by what she went through and I can't believe that she is *me*. I survived that, and I am here to tell the tale. Yet, my brain can't seem to put two and two together; it feels like I'm self plagiarizing a life story that isn't mine to share.

Even though it was clear that I was sick at this point, we still didn't know exactly what was wrong with me, and we wouldn't find out until I was able to see my new neurologist. Mom and I went to the hospital and did exactly what Dr. W advised us to do; when we told the Release of Information representative that we wanted every last medical document recorded under my name, she guffawed before realizing that we were dead serious.

It took a few weeks of back and forth before it was finally delivered…over 1,000 pages documenting every yearly checkup, stuffy nose, and UTI I'd had in my 16 years of life. Along with every appointment under Dr. E, the woman who diagnosed me with Conversion Disorder at age 13 and had been handling my care ever since.

If you've ever gone through a similar process, you may be wondering, how much did that cost? How in the world could you afford such a thing? We couldn't, not really. The hospital where my new neurologist was working offered to foot the bill and have us mail the records to them so they could start familiarizing themselves with my medical history before my first appointment. Now that I am able to reflect back on this experience, I realize how insanely privileged I was to have so many people on my side and eager to give me the medical attention I needed. *I only had to wait 3 years!*

Despite everything she put us through, mom and I felt it would be best to break up with Dr. E in person. We would have one last appointment where we could eviscerate her with the evidence we gathered, and then leave her behind, exposed and ashamed…that was the plan, at least. My misdiagnosis was not an accident; it was a coverup that was facilitated by multiple doctors with equivalent intentions.

When I recount my experiences under the care of these physicians, I truly feel as though they were waiting for me to either die or off myself before anyone found out the information they were hiding. It's not an easy thing to stomach. When the truth was revealed, Dr. E was probably shitting bricks, but I know that there was not even a skidmark of guilt on her conscience.

"Well," the doctor said as she opened the door, "we sure have a lot to discuss!" She smiled at us wildly like a cartoon rabid hyena.

I can't really remember what happened next, but at some point, I must have realized that we weren't going to get out of this without a fight, so I laid my iPod face down in my lap and began to record the interaction. Texas is a one-party consent state, which makes this completely legal. This is a transcription of the video, which is 4 minutes and 13 seconds long:

Mom: *[laughs]* her records are really nice.

Me: *[unintelligible]*

Mom: No no, no, don't even go there right now, okay? Everything that we told y'all– that it's been going on since the fifth grade– y'all put 'five months' instead of two and a half years. We have all of this on records. So, you know, we…we know what we told. My husband was there, and a few doctors have noted– I have it noted back in 2011– that we were telling them about this problem. So, uh…y– you're telling us that you called them and told them…

Dr. E: Called them and told them what?

Mom: …that you called the insurance company that we needed more physical therapy, doesn't dispute– it doesn't do anything for what they say Conversion Disorder needs, how long it should be for–

Dr. E: But that's– that's not–

Mom: Because Conversion Disorder–

Dr. E: That's not her diagnosis.

Me: *[talking over her]* So, why haven't you gotten rid of it?

Dr. E: I–

Mom; Because, you haven't told us anything except 'Conversion Disorder'.

Dr. E: No, that's not true!

Mom: When my husband was here, he asked you about conversion disorder…

Dr. E: We– we had–

Mom: …and you said 'I'm not ready to change that yet'

Dr. E: No, I didn't. That's not what I said.

Mom: Ivy, did she say she wasn't ready–

Me: That's ABSOLUTELY what you said.

Dr. E: *[stammering]* W-what I said…

Mom: *[scoffs]* Wow. Okay, you know what?

Me: You said that I have Conversion Disorder and a "separate" problem.

Mom: I don't see the point in talking when you won't even admit to what you said. Wow.

Dr. E: So, all the, um…*[pause]*

Mom: Wow. I have your records…

Me: Why are you smiling? Is this funny to you? You don't look like you're taking us seriously. You're smirking!

Dr. E: Well, I– this is not funny. This is very serious.

Mom: …four days before the neuropathy was found, you said she had no weakness, no pain, no nothing. Your records show that you noted that there is nothing wrong with her at all. No gait problem, no weakness…your records show that!

Dr. E: She– she has a gait problem because…

Me: Then why did you put that I didn't?

Mom: Why did you put that she didn't? Ivy, let's go.

Me: We have the medical records. You can deny till you die…I'm not stupid. I am NOT stupid.

Mom: We will be getting a new neurologist, this is ridiculous.

Dr. E: Ivy! You have small cell, small fiber neuropathy.

Mom: That's what you *think*. You think that, because you are just now starting to do tests. It was 2013 when you first saw her and said 'this is Conversion Disorder, I don't want to see her'. That– *[redacted primary care physician]* and you got together and decided that you were going to cover up the fact that she hadn't said anything for two and a half years. You think we can't see it? I have every bit of her medical records, every bit of them! I have some doctors that told the truth, and I have some doctors that didn't. So, Ivy, please...let's go.

Dr. E: Wait.

Mom: We are trying to get in with a new neurologist, and hopefully we can, because this is ridiculous. My husband sat right here when you said that you were not ready to change this [diagnosis].

Dr. E: That's not– That is not what I intended to communicate.

Mom: That is exactly what you said!

Me: Alright, Hilary Clinton. *[laughs]*

Mom: Yeah, exactly. Thank you.

Dr. E: Please…please don't leave, okay? Ivy? *[places hands on either arm rest of my chair]*

Me: Let me go. I don't– you've done enough. Please, let go of my wheelchair.

Mom: Please let go of her chhair. We are leaving NOW. You are refusing to let us leave?

Dr. E: No, I–

Mom: *[shouting]* excuse me, nurses, can you please help us leave this office? Please? The doctor is blocking the door!

Dr. E: I'm not…

Mom: Please open the door so I can leave!

Dr. E: You have a small fiber neuropathy…

Mom: You don't know what she has yet. Please open the door.

Dr. E: We have done thousands of tests!

Mom: Really? Please open the door.

Me: Your services are no longer needed.

Dr. E: You have small fiber neur–

Me: I know I have a problem! I've been telling you that for years! Please, let me get by. You've done enough.

Dr E: Ivy, listen…

Mom: You're blocking the door. I'm going– I'm going down to complain right now.

***

After we left the neurology clinic, Dr. E followed us out into the hallway, frantically spewing "Ivy, you have to listen to me, I want to help!"

All of the staff took shelter in place and watched the harassment happening in front of them; not a single person tried to help us leave. We got onto the elevator and the doctor squeezed her way in before the door could shut. Mom started to hyperventilate as Dr. E grabbed my chair again, saying "I want to help you, Ivy. You can't let her make you leave. You need to come with me!"

I forcefully pushed past her on the first floor and mom began pushing my chair speedily, unable to regulate her breathing. We turned a corner and found ourselves face to face with an aloof looking guy in a security uniform. Mom let out a sigh of relief before saying "Please, we need help, this woman is trying to prevent us from leaving". The security worker raised his brows at us and directed his gaze towards Dr. E, asking "Is there a problem here? Do you need me to escort them out of the building?"

Mom recoiled in shock and spat out *"We* need help!" between staggered gasps for air. Dr. E waved the security guard off like a pesky fart, telling him "Nothing to worry about. I just wanted to make sure this woman and her daughter found their way to human resources".

We did file a report about the minor hostage situation and placed an official complaint against Dr. E that day. The patient representatives expressed dubious concern and told us that an official investigation would be launched.

These are the progress notes written by Dr. E after the visit:

***

Progress Note:
[Redacted], MD at 6/9/2016
Author: *[Redacted]*, MD
Filed: 6/11/2016 3:44 PM
Editor: *[Redacted]*, MD (Physician)
Encounter Date: 6/9/2016
Author Type: Physician
Status: Signed

Ivy is a 16 yo. female seen for follow up in the Pediatric Neurology clinic today with her mother for Peripheral Neuropathy.

INTERVAL HISTORY:

Ivy reports that she initially got some relief of pain in her legs/feet with Lyrica but the past few weeks she has not been feeling well because she gets these "rushes of feeling dizzy and nauseous then hot". She feels if she can eat something it helps the symptoms pass, but she doesn't feel like it could be low blood sugar because she is eating meals and not skipping. Ivy and her mother reported that she is on hold for PT as the insurance has her listed as conversion disorder and they will not give many sessions for that diagnosis. I informed them that the PT request was submitted by me as peripheral neuropathy and I will call again to see what the delay is as I feel PT is very important for Ivy to become ambulatory. The mother reports they have an appointment with Neurology at *[redacted]* next month.

The mother became increasingly agitated at this point and said that she has seen all of the medical records and I have ruined her daughter's life for five years and I keep lying about everything because I diagnosed her with conversion disorder. Ivy and her mother wanted to leave the visit, as the mom has been agitated at prior visits but after talking for a few minutes we have a productive visit, I asked them to stay to discuss their concerns and to review what I tried to communicate at the most recent visit.

Ivy and the mother demanded to leave the room so I opened the door and accompanied them to the elevator and rode the elevator with them. The mother wanted to see *[redacted]* (Patient Relations) so I was walking her to the Patient Relations area and the mom was becoming increasingly agitated so I asked two staff members in the hall to accompany Ivy and her mother to Patient Relations.

REVIEW OF SYSTEMS (ROS): Not done as visit was terminated by pt and mom.
***

After this whole debacle, we still had one more test we had scheduled before I completely switched over to a new team of doctors. Think back to before the EMG was ordered, when my primary care physician ordered an MRI of my brain, going against Dr. E and her wishes…this was the second MRI of my brain, ever. The *first* one was done in 2013 when I was diagnosed with Conversion Disorder. Here are the results of the second scan, copy and pasted from MyChart:
***

Addendum

Please note, the mild posterior periventricular white matter signal abnormality is not new or changed since the prior examination.

Please change IMPRESSION #1 to read:

1. Stable appearance of mild bilaterally symmetric increased T2/FLAIR signal in posterior
periventricular white matter may represent remote insult v. abnormality of myelination;
clinical correlation recommended.

Discussed with Dr. [Redacted] at 2:00 p.m. on 5/16/2016.
Signed by [Redacted] on 05/17/2016 2:10 PM

IMPRESSION:

1. Bilaterally symmetric increased T2/FLAIR signal in posterior periventricular white matter may represent remote insult v. abnormality of myelination; clinical correlation recommended.
2. Large mucous retention cyst v. polyp remains present in the sphenoid sinus, and small mucous retention cyst v. polyp in right maxillary sinus; **both unchanged in the 2 1/2 year interval.**
3. Otherwise normal brain MRI with and without contrast.

***

I urge you to pay close attention to that little *addendum*. The 2016 scans of my brain showed white matter signal abnormality that was "not new" or changed since the last time an MRI was done of my brain...this is so tremendously important to remember, given the results of my previous MRI done 3 years earlier:

MRI BRAIN W WO CONTRAST
Collected on November 5, 2013 4:57 PM
Exam: MRI brain without and with contrast.
 Clinical history: Abnormal gait.

Findings:

MRI of the brain was performed using sagittal T1, axial T1, axial T2, axial FLAIR, axial gradient echo, coronal T1, and diffusion-weighted sequences with ADC mapping. 11.4 ml of Magnevist was administered and the T1-weighted sequences were repeated. The ventricles and cortical sulci are normal size, contour, and appearance. No parenchymal abnormality is noted. No extra-axial masses or collections are seen. The pituitary gland, optic chiasm, corpus callosum, and craniocervical junction demonstrate no abnormality.

Limited evaluation of the orbits and paranasal sinuses demonstrate a mucus retention cyst or polyp in the sphenoid sinus. Normal flow void is visualized in the internal carotid and vertebro-basilar systems. Examination of the diffusion-weighted images demonstrate no evidence of restricted diffusion. Examination of the postcontrast images demonstrate no abnormal enhancement.

Impression:

1. Normal MRI of the brain.

***

This diagnostic scan was reported as 100% "normal". Yet, the findings of this scan are identical to the findings of my 2016 scan, which showed abnormalities that suggested demyelination which would warrant "clinical correlation". They knew I was sick from the very beginning. Not only did they misdiagnose me, but, they withheld vital information about my health and neglected to treat me.

If you're reading all of this thinking, *why? What was the motivation behind such an elaborate scheme?*

The truth is: I have no idea. The scariest part about what happened to me is that there was no clear or reasonable motive. I was not treated as a human– a child– I was treated as a malignant wart that was stuck to the back of their minds. They let me grow more and more sick and ignored the problem for as long as they could. I am not special; this could happen to anyone. It happens to innocent people every single day. I am simply lucky enough to have made it out alive and to have the ability to tell my story.

Chapter 18

So, what was the *official* diagnosis? I would love to report that I was diagnosed with MS and that my new neurologist solved all of my problems immediately, that everything unfolded beautifully and I could finally live in peace…but that just wouldn't be *juicy* enough!

After my initial appointment with the neurology team on call that day, Dr. L looked at me with a furrowed brow, telling us "There is definitely something going on here, I would like to admit her for further examination". I concentrated on analyzing him– his mannerisms, rather than his actual words– as he spoke, not noticing how I was preemptively on the defense.

"What do you mean 'admit' me? Like, you want me to stay in the hospital?" I asked cautiously.

"Well, that would be the best course of action, in my opinion. I want to start from square one, essentially, and have you seen by a bunch of different specialists.

We are going to need to order a *lot* of tests" the doctor told me, sensing my growing anticipation.

I turned towards my parents and gave them that look you pull when you're trying to convince your mom to let you sleep over at a friend's house; desperately giddy, begging intensely. Mom and dad exchanged a nervous glance before mom spoke, saying "Okay, I also think that would be best. When exactly would we be doing this?"

There weren't any rooms available on the neurology floor at that very moment, so we went home and returned five days later as soon as a spot opened up. My father stayed back at home and continued going to work while mom and I stayed in the hospital, four hours away, for the next two weeks. I was 16 years old at this time, and I'll admit that I have little to no recollection of this specific stay at my current age of 23.

I was seen by multiple specialists outside of neurology, like rheumatology and infectious disease. They took an ungodly amount of blood for testing, leaving no stone unturned. They did *every test under the sun*, moon, and stars. I finally got my lumbar puncture, which came back mostly normal, besides showing elevated protein levels. They did a chest x-ray to check for sarcoidosis, and everything looked clean. I had to redo the EMG study and that wound up confirming the fact that I have nerve damage, but my muscles were unaffected. They did an MRI of my brain and spine using their "superior" equipment; apparently the images I had done before were subpar, like the difference between using an Andriod and an iPhone. These are the results we got:

***

MRI SPINE SCREENING WO/W CONTRAST
Addendum
Signed by [Redacted], MD on 7/28/2016 2:49 PM
These are not the classic appearances of NMO.
Impression:
Apparent T1 shortening returned from the periphery of the spinal cord following the administration of gadolinium, in the absence of precontrast T1-weighted imaging of the cervical and thoracic spine.

Appearances could represent evidence for inflammatory disorder versus prominent veins . Concern is raised for more diffuse abnormality of the spinal cord itself. Correlation with CSF is recommended. In addition precontrast imaging of the cervical and thoracic spine is recommended

EXAM: MRI CERVICAL, THORACIC AND LUMBAR SPINE WITH AND WITHOUT CONTRAST.

CLINICAL HISTORY: hyperreflexia

TECHNIQUE: Multiplanar multisequence MRI of the cervical, thoracic and lumbar spine was performed without and with intravenous contrast.

FINDINGS: There is some degradation of image quality owing to patient motion.

There appears to be a mild scoliosis bowed convex to the right of midline with its apex at the thoracolumbar junction.

There is apparent abnormal enhancement returned in a spotty pattern of distribution from the periphery of the spinal cord with multifocal punctate areas of apparent T1 shortening outlining most of the cervical and thoracic spine down to the level of the conus on postcontrast imaging without precontrast exam of the cervical or thoracic spine. A similar appearance to the lumbar spine is noted on the outside examination. No prominent vascular malformation identified

There is a normal complement of vertebral bodies.

There is normal alignment of the cervical, thoracic and lumbar spine.

The vertebrae and intervertebral discs have normal signal and morphology.

The spinal cord itself is without evidence for compression, expansion or atrophy..

The conus medullaris terminates in normal position at the mid body of L1. There is no thickening or fatty mass of the filum. The cauda equina is unremarkable.

MRI BRAIN AND ORBITS WO/W CONTRAST

Addendum

Signed by [Redacted], MD on 8/1/2016 5:46 PM

Comparison is now made to remote studies that have been uploaded and demonstrate presence of punctate enhancing foci in the brainstem as well as the cervical spine, which are more difficult to appreciate on the current exam owing to patient motion.

Differential diagnosis includes Clipper disease. Vasculitis and infection to include tick borne diseases are included in the differential.

These findings were discussed with [Redacted] on Friday 7/29/2016

Impression:

Mild diffuse volume loss with ringing in abnormal signal returned from the corpus callosum and periventricular white matter T2 hyperintensity best demonstrated on axial FLAIR imaging in addition to tiny multifocal punctate areas of T2 hyperintensity predominantly returned from the bilateral prefrontal lobes without evidence for breakdown of the blood brain barrier. Appearances are unchanged when compared to the outside study performed 5/13/2016 and consistent with remote insult.

Apparently intact optic pathways without radiographic evidence for optic neuritis at this time.

Mucous retention cyst and partial opacification of the mastoid air cells as described

Please see also same day report of MR lumbar spine complete with postcontrast imaging of the whole spine

EXAM: MRI BRAIN AND ORBITS WITH AND WITHOUT CONTRAST.

CLINICAL HISTORY: Blurry vision, spastic paraparesis in a 16-year-old female

TECHNIQUE: Multiplanar multisequence MRI of the brain and orbits was performed without and with intravenous contrast.

FINDINGS: There is some degradation of image quality following the administration of gadolinium due to patient motion.

Optic nerves, chiasm and tracts are normal in size and signal. There is no abnormality involving the globes, extraocular muscles or other intraorbital structures. There is no intraorbital mass or pathologic enhancement. There is no sellar nor suprasellar mass.

There is some generalized volume loss both above and below the tentorium with widening of the extra-axial CSF spaces and sulci. No discrete extra-axial collection is seen. No mass lesions identified.

On the sagittal T1-weighted midline imaging there are at least 2 discrete foci of T1 shortening without clearly associated enhancement returned from the frontal and occipital diploic spaces. The body of the corpus callosum appears generally thinned.

The supratentorial ventricular system is minimally prominent with some apparent periventricular T2 hyperintensity best seen on axial flair imaging. In particular the temporal horns retain normal morphology and hippocampi appear to return symmetric signal bilaterally

There are multifocal tiny punctate nonenhancing T2 hyperintensities returned from the bifrontal white matter.

There are no regions of restricted diffusion. No altered blood or blood product demonstrated on gradient echo imaging

There is no pathologic intracranial contrast enhancement. The right superior ophthalmic vein is noted to be more prominent than its companion on the left.

Expected flow voids are demonstrated in the arteries about the circle of Willis.

The paranasal sinuses demonstrate a mucous retention cyst within the left sphenoid loculus. There is partial opacification of the right greater than left-sided mastoid air cells.

***

I had spent the last 3 years of my life dreaming of the day a doctor would look me in the eyes sympathetically and say, *"We know what's wrong with you. The answer was so obvious!"* Dr. L stood with his brow furrowed even more than the day I met him with a team of bright-eyed residents in the background, eager to learn. He told us that I was considered an 8 on the EDSS scale, which is described as "Essentially restricted to bed or chair or pushed in wheelchair. May be out of bed itself much of the day. Retains many self-care functions. Generally has effective use of arms" (Multiple Sclerosis Trust).

After reviewing the details of every last test with several physicians within the hospital and across the country at the Mayo Clinic, Dr. L was ready to issue a new diagnosis that would remain tentative until we saw how I reacted to treatment: I was diagnosed with CLIPPERS disease.

Rather than feeling a rush of relief, I just sat there feeling equally as stuck. "Um, I'm sorry, I've never heard of that one," I said sheepishly.

I spent countless hours researching all the possible diseases that I might have based on my symptoms, and I was truly expecting to hear a familiar name pop up. Dr. L gave me a hesitant chuckle and responded "Well, I've only ever seen one other pediatric case of it before. This disease is fairly new, the medical literature on CLIPPERS only goes back to around 2010".

So…what is CLIPPERS? This is an acronym for chronic lymphocytic inflammation with pontine perivascular enhancement responsive to steroids.

Chronic lymphocytic inflammation with pontine perivascular enhancement responsive to steroids (CLIPPERS) is an autoimmune-mediated disease that causes my body to attack my central nervous system, which has left me with swelling in my brain and spine. It's characterized by radiographic findings of a "spotty" or "peppered" pattern throughout the pons and spinal cord; imagine what it might look like if you sneezed and left behind a splattering of dispersed dots, where each dot is an area of active inflammation. The RS, standing for "responsive to steroids", is specifically important because the disease has typically proven to show vast improvement after steroid therapy.

I remained hesitant and outwardly dubious of this diagnosis, because it didn't feel "fair". I waited so long for a final conclusion, only to be told that I have a rare disease that came with more questions than answers. The doctors had to take a "learn as you go" approach with my treatment. I was approached by dozens of medical research students who I permitted to use my scans and other test results in studies about various other demyelinating, autoimmune-mediated diseases (including MS).

I would repeatedly request a prognosis for my disease, and each time Dr. L would become uncomfortable and tell me that he simply couldn't predict such a thing. There was a huge part of me that wished I was diagnosed with something "easy" like cancer, because everyone knows what that is, and we have more than enough knowledge on how to treat the many, specific versions of it. I wanted clear, concrete answers.

One of the rheumatology doctors who followed along with my treatment suggested I try creating a Facebook group for other people with CLIPPERS, because there's a community for everything on the internet, right? Through my own amateur Google searches, there seem to only be 10 reported cases of pediatric-onset CLIPPERS worldwide, with "The mean age at onset [being] 50 years (range 13 to 86 years)" (NCBI).

The exact timeline of treatments I did over the years is fuzzy for me, but I can assure you that we basically went down the line of all the most prevalent treatment routes for autoimmune diseases. I was initially started with a 5 day round of IV prednisone, doing 1000 milligrams a day. There are no words I can think of to describe the horrors of roid rage…one time I wanted to get a rootbeer from the fridge, as this was one of the few things that would help alleviate the constant taste of poison that coated my mouth. When my brother told me that he had taken the last one, I sat in the bathroom and cried for 3 hours while I genuinely contemplated killing myself. It was scarily miserable.

The goal has always been to find a "steroid-sparing agent", meaning, a treatment that I could take along with (or in place of) steroids. Long-term steroid use can have some nasty effects on the body, but, so can CLIPPERS…it's a fun game of "which outcome sounds worse?" In 2018 they did a brain biopsy where they took a tissue sample from one of the lesions, and I was told that this confirmed the presence of CLIPPERS.

I underwent a second brain biopsy in 2020, mostly for my own peace of mind; my health was declining enough that Dr. L felt it was justifiable to "double-check", but he warned me that the results would likely come back the same as the first time. This is what they documented after the second biopsy:

Immunophenotyping of the infiltrating lymphocytes shows a predominance of CD8 positive cells and is consistent with an immune-mediated process. Although the epicenter appears based in the white matter, there is also some involvement of the gray matter. No. infectious organism is seen. No viral inclusions or evidence of virus specific cytopathic effect is seen. Morphologicallly similar to previous biopsy.

I was always very untrusting and verbally combative with all of my doctors, which I harbor a lot of guilt about now. I found myself suffering from the "Truman Show Effect", which resulted in me lashing out and doubting almost everything that came out of my doctors' mouths. The second brain biopsy showed identical results to the first.

By the time I reached the age of 22, I could tell that Dr. L was exasperated and defeated. What started out as an exciting mystery, jigsaw puzzle of a case, became a never-ending pit of dead ends and unexplainable conundrums. Even with medical science evolving and bringing us new discoveries every day, there simply hasn't been enough time passed for us to have a coherent understanding of CLIPPERS as a disease. We are still learning how best to treat it, and what exactly causes it in the first place.

I'm now being seen by all adult providers at the *geriatric* age of 23, and the switch that finally cut off all ties to pediatrics made me feel like I was being given a fresh start. I no longer have any reason to step foot in the hospital where I was originally diagnosed with conversion disorder. I don't have to worry about providers turning me away because of my age. I no longer have to fight to get people to believe me, and my parents aren't the first source of information my doctors turn to.

I am Ivy Babbitt, I'm 23 years old (currently), and I have a disease called CLIPPERS. I was misdiagnosed with Conversion Disorder from ages 13-16. My treatment consists of mostly trial and error and is ongoing. I cannot wait to see where the research regarding CLIPPERS is at 10 years from now. I am disabled in ways that are likely permanent, and I am at peace with this reality. After fighting for so long to be heard, I am now focusing on living my day-to-day life in a way that brings me joy and fulfillment.

I'm in therapy to work through my traumatic past, which has immensely improved my self-image and the way I approach interpersonal relationships. I've been fostering cats and kittens since 2020, and it has changed my life so dramatically; the youngest foster I've had was less than 24 hours old, and I have found that I specifically love the "orphan", singleton bottle-babies. Also, I wrote a book!

I still have an entire greenhouse worth of growing to do, but I choose to trust the process and keep moving forward.

www.ingramcontent.com/pod-product-compliance
Lightning Source LLC
Chambersburg PA
CBHW051043250726
48656CB00001B/119